Medicine and the Marketplace

Medicine and the Marketplace

The Moral Dimensions of Managed Care

KENMAN L. WONG

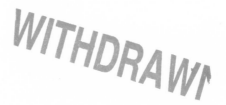

University of Notre Dame Press

NOTRE DAME, INDIANA

Library of Congress Cataloging-in-Publication Data

Wong, Kenman L., 1964–
    Medicine and the marketplace : the moral dimensions of managed
care / Kenman L. Wong.
        p.   cm.
    Includes bibliographical references and index.
    ISBN 0–268–01440–X (alk. paper)
    1. Managed care plans (Medical care)—Moral and ethical aspects.
2. Medical care—Moral and ethical aspects.   3. Health care
rationing—Moral and ethical aspects.   4. Medical ethics—Standards.
I. Title.
RA413.W67   1999
362.1'04258—dc21   98–30622

Contents

Preface

This book is an outcome of the pressing need for ethical reflection on the changing nature of the American health care system, particularly the role and responsibilities of large-scale organizations. Each of the significant stakeholders in medicine, including health care professionals, patients, health plan administrators, insurance companies, and the broader society, is faced with new and complex moral challenges. While much focus has been given to the dilemmas that physicians are facing at the bedside, there has been a lack of substantive inquiry into the ethics of the organizations whose practices and policies contribute to the quandaries health care providers face.

The goal of this book is to shed light on these important topics by examining a number of important questions, including the following: Can organizations engaged in the task of profit-making properly honor the interests of patients? Will physicians under contract to managed care plans be faced with divided loyalties, leading to harm to patients? Should the profit motive play any role in medicine?

These are critical questions for which facile answers will not suffice. As the reader will see, I am not convinced that the solution to the dilemmas arising at the new intersections of business and medicine is to jettison managed care outright. Such proposals are much too simple. Managed care is not intrinsically evil. However, the policies used to determine the way care is delivered have the potential to cause great harm. Thus, the ethical values behind policy and procedure setting must be rigorously examined and reformulated if these new health care arrangements are to guard the interests of patients and providers. In the following pages, I will focus on these issues and develop ideas so that managed care can become an ethics-driven system.

The completion of a project of this nature requires the work of many hands. I am deeply indebted to a number of people who have made substantive intellectual contributions to this book. William W. May, John P. Crossley, and Ian I. Mitroff of the University of Southern California and Scott B. Rae of the Talbot School of Theology deserve particular mention as scholars who gave insightful guidance and editorial suggestions on earlier versions of this manuscript. I am also indebted to a number of health care professionals. In the formal settings in which I have presented ideas from this book, and in personal encounters, they have provided priceless firsthand insights into the changing nature of medicine.

I am also appreciative of the efforts of staff members at the University of Notre Dame Press, in particular, Director James Langford and Editor Rebecca DeBoer. Jim clearly saw the vision behind this project and offered insightful editorial guidance along the way. Calling Rebecca's editing work remarkable is a great understatement. Her eye for details and suggestions for changes on the manuscript have truly been invaluable.

In addition to intellectual challenges, writing can be a lonely task. Good relationships are necessary to reduce the sense of isolation that is often the by-product of solitary days spent in front of a computer screen. I am very thankful to dedicated friends, family members, and colleagues (past and present) who have helped to provide a sense of "community" during the course of this project.

Finally, and most importantly, I am especially appreciative of the efforts of my wife, Marika. In addition to her superb editorial work on earlier versions of the manuscript, her courage, patience, and love have been of heroic proportions during the time I have devoted to this project. Despite a highly demanding schedule, she has consistently found the strength to be an attentive listener and source of wisdom and encouragement. On many days when I felt overwhelmed by this endeavor, she gently reminded me of the greater purposes to which we are working together. It is to her, and our newborn son, Callan, that this work is gratefully dedicated.

Introduction

Recent headlines have raised significant levels of public concern over the emerging dominance of managed health care, particularly when it is delivered by corporations engaged in the quest for financial gains for shareholders.[1] A number of real-life cases have highlighted the ethical dilemmas which can arise when the profit motive of business is mixed with the healing mission of medicine. Patients allegedly have been harmed or placed at serious risk as a direct result of various cost-cutting practices adopted to improve the bottom line.

Several observers point out that vexing moral dilemmas pitting profit against patient interests are inevitable since managed care organizations are, by their very nature, placed in a moral bind. These institutions have conflicting roles in their attempt to function both as traditional businesses, which have financial obligations to shareholders, and as medical entities, which have duties to uphold the best interests of patients.[2]

When these two obligations conflict, the fear is that pecuniary interests will prevail, harming patients and eroding the moral substance of medicine in the process. For instance, Lonnie Bristow, former president of the American Medical Association, stated in an interview:

> We now have health care being controlled by MBA's rather than by physicians committed to the Hippocratic Oath . . . once health care becomes corporatized . . . then its major commitment is to Wall Street and the stockholders to maximize profits, rather than to give the best possible patient care. Business principles are introduced that unfortunately put patient care second to corporate profits.[3]

While these types of sentiments about the new intersections of business and medicine have become popular, managed care is not without numerous supporters, including many members of the medical profession. Citing the positive effects on health care costs, advocates of managed care argue that despite a few headlining cases, marketplace discipline works to better serve societal interests than the older fee-for-service model.[4] Under the dominance of this earlier approach, there were few incentives to limit expenditures, since third-party insurers usually paid the bills without much scrutiny. It is well-documented that this approach led to greatly overprescribed medical procedures. This contributed to a climate of rising costs, which in turn helped deny access to insurance coverage for millions of Americans. In contrast, market competition through managed care seems an auspicious method to reverse these trends, since it uses incentives which promise to simultaneously reduce costs and improve quality and access.[5]

Managed care has had some success in stabilizing costs, but there are also suspicions that its success has been achieved at the direct expense of patient health. Persistent and crucial questions surround the ethics of managed care and the behavior of the organizations involved in its delivery. Foremost, many wonder whether or not managed care is the proper direction for medical delivery reform, particularly since its cost-savings mechanisms alter the traditional patient-physician relationship.[6] Simply put, how can physicians fulfill their role as patient advocate when these newer incentive systems reward them for controlling costs?

Furthermore, even if managed care is determined to be preferable to other alternatives, should profit-seeking organizations be engaged in its delivery?[7] If not, managed care will be the exclusive domain of non-profit organizations. Yet non-profit institutions also compete and engage in other "business" activities. For example, they also must hold the line on expenses, earn profits in the form of "surpluses" in order to finance growth, and market their services to attract subscribers. If for-profits as well as non-profits are acceptable, what type of an ethical framework should guide these organizations so that patient interests are properly protected against financial goals? A traditional business approach with its focus on profit maximization is inadequate, while a traditional medical model may be unsound fiscally, and ignores the commercial aspects and obligations of managed care institutions.

LIMITATIONS OF THE CURRENT DEBATE

Concerns of this nature have led to a host of normative ethical opinions from both scholarly and popular sources. However, much of what has been expressed so far oversimplifies the debate. This severely impedes a proper assessment of the morality of managed care and the development of ethical standards.

To begin with, the debate is often cast as a simple dichotomy, pitting managed care against fee-for-service medicine. While some of those who are opposed to the newer system advocate a return to more traditional arrangements, and while managed care is clearly replacing fee-for-service as the dominant model, the dichotomy is misleading. A number of critics of managed care favor other methods of reform which claim to address the moral as well as the financial shortcomings of fee-for-service medicine. For example, proposals have been advanced in support of explicit rationing models, such as the recent Oregon plan, in order to ensure fairness in the distribution of medical resources. Other proposals favor the use of Medical Savings Accounts to create patient autonomy and to unleash true free-market reforms in order to reduce costs. In light of these options, a comprehensive moral assessment of managed care must be conducted in the context of these and other major alternatives, not just of fee-for-service arrangements.

Similarly, a simplistic form of the debate mistakenly categorizes all those who advocate managed care arrangements as proponents of *laissez-faire* medicine. While supporters of managed care do share many arguments in common, a number simultaneously reject a "free market" approach to medicine. For instance, some favor these arrangements but with greater legal protections for patients and physicians than those that industry representatives publicly support. Moreover, some support the principles and goals behind managed care but argue, on moral grounds, that it must be delivered through the exclusive use of non-profit organizations. Clearly, these perspectives also need to be brought into the discussion.

Other efforts at conducting the debate place all of the respective "critics" and "supporters" of managed care in polar opposition.[8] While I will also initially cast the discussion in these terms because it is useful for purposes of an introduction to the issues, such a simple opposition is inadequate. It encourages the assumption that the respective supporters and critics of managed care are univocal. It also permits "critics" to express purely destructive forms of criticism against managed care without spelling out concrete alternatives for reform.[9] The interview including the earlier-cited statement by former AMA president Bristow is a case in point. Bristow attacks managed care, especially when for-profit organizations are involved, but fails to articulate a positive prescription for change. This lack of a concrete alternative for reform can lead the public to the erroneous conclusion that the solution to ethical dilemmas in medical delivery is the abolition of managed care. When all the available alternatives to managed care are delineated and scrutinized, it becomes evident that the answer is not so simple.

Another significant weakness of much of the current debate is that it has been predominantly focused on the ethical implications of changes in the patient-physician relationship. As a result, the burden has been almost exclusively placed on the shoulders of doctors to resolve these ongoing ethical dilemmas. Physicians are told, as a matter of law and ethics, that despite threats to their financial well-being, they are to remain in the role of ideal patient advocate.[10]

While the values of individual physicians undoubtedly play a critical role in clinical decision making, the organizations involved also wield tremendous amounts of power to shape the context in which ethical challenges arise. They play an important part in creating cultures that influence physician practices. Yet, aside from simplistic depictions of "greedy corporations," issues of business ethics have been, until very recently, almost ignored in the debate. Susan Wolf has commented on the dearth of scholarly effort on organizational ethics in health care that incorporates the work that already exists in corporate ethics.[11] As she points out:

we have been left with a myopia that most ethical problems can and should be resolved by the individual treating physician . . . In the domain of organizational ethics, we know even less. The formulation of ethics for health care organizations is in its infancy. We need both to press for a rich substantive vision of institutional ethics and to analyze and compare organizational knowledge and behavior with any such vision.[12]

Contributing to this lack of an investigative overlap with corporate ethics is a natural aversion to "business" in the medical community. Many health care practitioners, reflecting the sentiments expressed by Bristow, have a strong antipathy toward business because of its presumed single-minded goal of maximizing profit. This is in direct contrast to their beliefs about the patient-centered orientation of medicine. Yet, the growth of enrollment in plans offered by for-profit corporations demands that these new intersections be investigated and that implications for organizational ethics be clearly defined. Ignoring these areas of overlap will only serve to exacerbate existing problems.

EXPANDING THE DEBATE

The overall aim of this book is to advance the managed care debate by conducting a comprehensive ethical assessment of the participation of for-profit organizations in managed care. Some of the shortcomings in the way the current debate has been shaped will be remedied. In particular, I will expand the simplistic two-part rubric—managed care vs. fee-for-service medicine—into a typology that more adequately takes into account the plurality of viewpoints which have been expressed on the subject of health care delivery. This typology will provide a framework for taking a critical look at the competing alternatives to managed care. A broader depiction of the debate will reveal that the solution to the dilemmas which have arisen is not a simple return to fee-for-service medicine.

This more comprehensive framework will also enable us to evaluate the moral viability of for-profit organizations in the delivery of managed care. This is a critical issue, since the argument that only non-profit organizations should be engaged in the delivery of this newer form of medicine is one of the primary focal points of the current discussion.[13]

Much has already been written on the responsibilities of individual physicians when they are faced with dilemmas that challenge their commitment to the well-being of their patients. However, as noted earlier, the discussion of institutional ethics is still in its infancy. Since organizations, especially those chartered as profit-seeking, are taking on an increasingly dominant role in health care, it is critical that their moral responsibilities, as *organizations*, be delineated.

To be sure, the development of ethics for these institutions is a difficult task, given their dual functions as both medical and business entities and the conflicting obligations these roles entail. In fact, some claim that it is all but impossible to reconcile these identities. When attempts have been made to develop such a framework in the past, it has very often been the case that only one of these functions has been included, resulting in the neglect of a host of important interests.[14] Consequently, a considerable amount of effort will be devoted to developing a governing moral paradigm for managed care organizations which accounts for both sets of obligations. From such a framework, we can delineate some of the specific moral responsibilities which can be assigned to managed care organizations and to some of the other most important stakeholders in the new health care environment.

The reader should know that several foundational premises underlie this book. First, the assumption is that fiscal resources for health care are limited. Thus, unless the decision is made on a societal level to allocate funds to cover health care procedures ad infinitum, there will continue to be a need to reform health care delivery so that costs are brought under control.

Second, the focus of this work is on health care *delivery*. The concept of "health care reform" raises images of the debate during the early years of the Clinton administration. The focus here is limited to questions over the reform of *delivery* rather than on aggregate level *financing*. Consequently, some of the issues raised during the Clinton administration's discussions, in which single-payer and employer-based "pay or play" financing options were considered, will not be addressed.

Although the issues surrounding financing and delivery through "managed competition" were conjoined during these discussions, they are separable to a large degree. For instance, regardless of which type of financing mechanism is employed, the tradeoffs with respect to delivery options must still be examined. Fee-for-service, managed care, various rationing plans, or Medical Savings Accounts could be used in conjunction with a single-payer or an employer-financed system. Uwe Reinhardt has insightfully divided these areas for reform into two categories: the "cash-intake" and "cash disbursement" facets of the health system.[15] This book's focus will be on the latter.

Third, an ethical assessment of managed care, as opposed to purely economic or medically based evaluations of it, must be based upon specific normative moral criteria. I will rely upon the well-known principles for justice set forth by John Rawls in his seminal work, *A Theory of Justice*.[16] Rawls derives his principles of justice through a fictitious "constitutional convention," in which the parties involved select principles to govern society while blinded to their own social positions behind a "veil of ignorance." In this thought experiment, no one can dominate based upon natural endowment or societal position because all are placed in an "original position." Rawls hypothesizes that the social contractors, while ignorant of their own particulars, will unanimously choose two principles to distribute social goods. The first principle requires that each person be permitted the greatest amount of liberty compatible with similar liberty for others. The second, known as the "difference principle," stipulates that once this basic liberty is guaranteed, inequalities in social goods will only be allowed if they benefit everyone, especially the "representative least-advantaged person" in society.

The foundation upon which Rawls bases his theory has received criticism, especially from communitarian and feminist thinkers who take issue with some of his assumptions about the nature of human beings in the "original position."[17] However, he accounts for many of these criticisms in his more recent work, *Political Liberalism*.[18] According to Rawls, his conception of persons in the "original position" is a political rather than a metaphysical or metaethical one. In addition, he allows for the possibility that complex persons with irreconcilable and incompatible particular perspectives can engage in the quest for a modest "reasonable pluralism" in a democratic society. With these adaptations, his theory is a much more plausible and useful tool for reaching some form of ethical consensus in a pluralistic society. His broad principles of justice are assumed in seeking consensus on the ethics of managed care.

Chapter 1, "Business and Medicine at a New Crossroads," provides an overview of the growth of managed care arrangements and a detailed description of the resulting ethical tensions at the level of both the individual physician and the organization. In addition, it describes the current legal and regulatory environment and points out specific areas in which ethical and social policy guidelines need to be further developed.

Chapter 2, "Reframing the Debate: Perspectives Critical of Managed Care," builds a typology which recasts and broadens the debate. As noted, most frame the debate as one in which there are only two perspectives. This limits the scope of a proper moral assessment and the development of appropriate ethical responsibilities and policy guidelines. Chapter 2 develops a six-part typology of the alternatives to health care delivery which are currently being advanced. This typology reveals that the debate is much more nuanced than a simple dichotomy. After developing this framework, chapter 2 presents a detailed description of the arguments offered by the three "types" who oppose managed care: those who favor a return to fee-for-service medicine, those who support the use of Medical Savings Accounts (MSAs), and those who suggest the use of explicit rationing models.

Chapter 3, "Reframing the Debate: Perspectives in Support of Managed Care," continues the work of the previous chapter. It presents the detailed arguments and policy proposals of the three "types" who support managed care: those who champion the use of free-market approaches, those who support only non-profit managed care organizations, and those who favor the concepts behind managed care, but with significant ethical and legal limits on specific organizational behavior.

Chapter 4, "Fee-For-Service Medicine," begins the process of evaluating the morality of the general concept of managed care. In particular, managed care is compared with the delivery model it is predominantly replacing, namely, fee-for-service arrangements. Chapter 4 concludes that managed care is a vastly superior approach to health care delivery.

Chapter 5, "Alternative Reform Proposals," continues the task of assessing the morality of managed care. In this chapter, managed care is compared with some newer reform proposals, namely, Medical Savings Accounts and explicit rationing programs. The conclusion is that while it is not necessarily a perfect solution, managed care is a morally superior method of medical delivery.

Chapter 6, "The Ethical Importance of the Non-Profit Distinction," assesses the accuracy of the claim that if managed care is the preferred option, only non-profit organizations should be engaged in its delivery since these institutions pose less of a threat to already tenuous patient-physician relationships. After engaging in a systematic comparison of the two models, chapter 6 argues that the differences between for-profit and non-profit institutions are largely overstated. Although there are *some* differences between the two models, these disparities do not justify the proscription of for-profit plans. In fact, when they are examined closely, there are many similarities between the two types of organizations.

Chapter 7, "The Moral Viability of For-Profit Organizations," examines the claim that the continued growth of for-profit organizations in the context of free-market competition should be encouraged, because these entities are best suited to the current health care environment. While this chapter will offer support for the involvement of profit-seeking organizations, it rejects the claim that only minimal restraints should be placed on these institutions because market forces will adequately govern their behavior.

Chapter 8, "Business Ethics for Managed Care Organizations," argues that a tenable case can be made on behalf of the morality of these institutions only if they are grounded in a more "enlightened" model of business. The disparities in the medical and business obligations of these organizations can be reduced if these institutions are held to substantive ethical standards, which work to ensure that patient health is not sacrificed for financial gain. Such a model also offers much promise in terms of forming guiding moral principles and social policies to ensure that managed care organizations are indeed serving society's best interests.

In developing this framework, chapter 8 draws upon some promising work in the field of business ethics which makes a strong case against the narrow "custodian of wealth" model of business, both in terms of its descriptive accuracy and its normative preferability. This chapter also addresses concerns that a business model, no matter how "enlightened," is inadequate to the task of governing health care organizations because the normative goals of business and medicine are simply too different. After responding to these concerns, chapter 8 offers several reasons why a reformulated business model is preferable to a traditional medical model, given the fiscal constraints in today's health care environment.

Chapter 9, "Stakeholder Responsibilities in the New Health Care Environment," describes the specific ethical obligations of managed care organizations which can be extracted from the framework developed in chapter 8. In addition, it delineates the responsibilities of the other important stakeholders in the new medical environment. These include the reciprocal responsibilities of the broader community, employers, and patients. Given these shared responsibilities, there is far less reason than many believe to fear the growth of managed health care and the involvement of for-profit organizations in its delivery. Managed care organizations can indeed operate in a manner that honors the interests of patients and the broader society.

One   Business and Medicine at a New Crossroads

The uneasy tension inherent in the pursuit of profit through the practice of medicine has long been the subject of public moral concern. Medical history is replete with controversies over fee-setting, the exercise of professional dominance to undermine competitors, and the presence of financial incentives to overprescribe health care procedures. These issues have attracted increasing interest during the last two decades due to concerns over the rate of escalation of health care costs. As a result, a host of scholarly studies have been conducted and a number of laws written to regulate some of the profit-seeking behavior of doctors.[1]

While abuses in the medical profession are undoubtedly troubling, some of the practices of managed care organizations also raise moral issues directly centered around the clash of the profit motive and patient well-being. Observers allege that these newer practices are more insidious and have the potential to create greater harm for patients than abuses of the past. However, despite tremendous resistance from some quarters of the medical profession, health care has rapidly evolved and profit-seeking organizations have become the dominant institutions engaged in the delivery of care.

BACKGROUND AND HISTORY

Managed care can be briefly characterized as a system that integrates the financing and delivery of health care by means of several key features.[2] First, managed care organizations contract with selected physicians and hospitals, who agree to furnish a comprehensive set of health care services to enrolled members, usually in exchange for either a fixed monthly premium or for reduced rates on a fee-for-service basis. Second, these providers (the "network") typically accept utilization and quality controls as a part of their contracts. Third, patients are given financial incentives to use these providers and facilities. Services rendered by "out-of-network" physicians or facilities are either not covered at all by the plan or come at a higher out-of-pocket cost to the patient than services rendered "in the network."

While this approach to health care has only recently become so dominant, the basic concept underlying managed care has been in existence in the United States since fraternal societies established prepaid medical care programs in 1787.[3] The current manifestation of the model had its genesis over fifty years ago, when prepaid group practices such as Kaiser-Permanente arose to provide cost-efficient health care to company employees.

Due to sharp increases in health care costs and resulting concerns about who would ultimately bear the cost, managed care began to gain significant prominence over two decades ago. The Nixon administration embraced prepaid group practice as its preferred policy for curbing the explosive growth of the nation's health care expenditures and worked with Democratic legislators to enact the Health Maintenance Organization Act of 1973.[4] In order to meet the aggressive goal of creating 1700 HMOs that could serve 40 million members by 1973, the federal government awarded subsidies of $200 million to non-profit groups to form organizations under this act.[5] Though the administration fell short of its numerical goals, HMOs nonetheless experienced tremendous growth.

The most significant increase of enrollment in such plans has occurred during the last ten years. By early 1997, membership had already grown to over 65 million nationwide, up from 36.5 million in 1990. Several forces have led to this dramatic expansion. One of the most powerful engines fueling the current growth in enrollment is the prompting of employers, who pay for all or at least a large portion of the health care benefits of most Americans. Most employers believe that managed care organizations are their best hope of keeping the prices on their costliest benefit in check. In the last decade, they have watched health insurance premiums evolve into the single largest contributor to their overhead costs.

This has also raised concerns about the negative effect on their ability to compete globally.

Further prompting the employers' need to control costs were new accounting laws requiring publicly-held companies to estimate future health care costs for retirees on balance sheets.[6] In order to curb these increasing financial demands, employers have encouraged enrollment in more cost-efficient managed care programs rather than traditional indemnity plans, sparking tremendous growth in the industry.

In addition to employer-related increases in enrollment, several other factors are contributing to the growth of these plans. An increasing fear, similar to but more pronounced than the concerns of two decades ago which prompted the initial growth of managed care, is that aggregate-level health care spending is spiraling out of control. Total U.S. health care expenditures were 13 percent of GNP in 1991, up from 9.1 percent in 1980, and expected to reach 15 percent by the year 2000.[7] More importantly, these numbers represent a widening spending gap between the U.S. and other countries, further contributing to concerns about eroding global competitiveness on a national level. Several well-documented trends have been identified as the primary contributors to the dramatic increase in expenditures. The most significant of these include expensive, rapidly developing technology, an aging population, the demand for miracle cures, and limitless demands for treatments to prolong life.

In response to these challenges, lawmakers continue to encourage managed care as a solution to runaway health care outlays. The concept was a critical component of the proposed national health care reform plan offered by the Clinton administration during his early years in office. More recently, Republican legislators have also been promoting enrollment in health maintenance organizations as one method of capping the amount spent annually on Medicare.[8]

Despite the well-intentioned beginnings of managed care and its continued support by government officials, several aspects of its expansion have become morally controversial. Of particular concern is the fact that the plans experiencing the most significant increases in enrollment are ones being offered by profit-seeking organizations. Managed care was once dominated by non-profit practices organized under a "staff model," and with a sense of social mission, like Kaiser-Permanente. Managed care as an "industry" is witnessing the rapid entry and success of shareholder-owned corporations. In 1988, for-profit plans had a total enrollment of 15.4 million members and non-profit plans had 17.2 million. By 1993, enrollment in for-profit plans had increased dramatically to 24.8 million, far surpassing the 20.4 million enrolled in non-profit plans.[9] By 1995, there were over 12 million members enrolled in managed care plans in the state of California alone, with approximately 7 million of these in plans sponsored by for-profit providers.[10] This has led some observers to state that managed care offered by for-profit organizations has already become *de facto* health policy.[11] In a more negative light, some physicians have expressed concern that "the dollar sign is replacing the caduceus" as the dominant symbol of medicine.[12]

NEW ETHICAL CHALLENGES

Given the business aspects of managed care organizations, many people in the broader public wonder if the growth of these plans, and their resulting profits, come at the direct expense of the well-being of patients. In direct contrast to the *over-prescription* problem of the past, the potential for ethical conflicts in managed care involves the possibility of patient harm due to the *under-prescription* of medical procedures. Given the fact that the utilization of health care procedures in prepaid arrangements can be a direct short-term expense against a plan and/or a physician's financial bottom line, the natural temptation is to withhold care.

Especially troubling are allegations that managed care organizations interfere in the physician-patient relationship through the use of financial incentives and other measures which induce doctors to *deny* necessary treatments in the quest for cost-containment and increased returns to shareholders. Under increasingly popular prepaid or "capitated" payment arrangements, individual doctors or hospitals agree to receive, in exchange for a set number of patients, a fixed monthly fee-per-enrollee from an MCO (managed care organization) independent of how many services are actually provided. The amount paid is supposed to cover the cost of office visits, additional procedures, and in some cases, specialty referrals. The physician or hospital under contract receives the same amount of payment regardless of whether the patient is a healthy enrollee who never visits the office during the year, or a sick enrollee requiring a significant amount of care.

In a typical arrangement, primary care physicians coordinate the patient's care and manage costs by acting as "gatekeepers" to other medical services. In order to receive expensive procedures or see specialists, patients must receive a referral from their primary care physician. Unlike traditional fee-for-service medicine, under which the insurer assumed all of the financial risk for cost overruns, managed care arrangements usually share this risk with physicians. In essence, doctors take on the same sort of risks as an insurance company, which hopes that the money it collects in the form of premiums will be more than the claims it must pay.

Under some contracts, physicians receive a percentage of their compensation based upon performance, which is often measured in economic terms. While this practice is not universal, the organizations which engage in it typically withhold from 12 to 20 percent of salary until the end of the year.[13] During this time, the actual costs for specialty referrals and hospitalizations are compared with revenues from the premiums allocated to cover these costs. If there is a deficit, the insurer keeps the amount withheld to cover the overruns. Conversely, if there is a surplus, the plan returns all or some of these funds to the physician. In some situations, more than the actual withheld amount is paid as a "bonus" for meeting cost-containment goals. Within these arrangements, it is evident that there is a built-in financial incentive, from a purely short-term economic standpoint, to expend only a limited amount of resources on each patient, since extra time, expensive procedures, or referral to specialists come directly out of the physician's own pocket.

Critics point to a recent well-publicized legal case in Southern California as a poignant illustration of the ethical challenges to doctors as a result of these arrangements. In this case, the family of thirty-four-year-old Joyce Ching filed a malpractice suit against her physician, Dr. Elvin C. Gaines, for her premature death from cancer. The suit alleged that Ching's medical care was adversely affected by Gaine's incentives to cut costs in order to increase his own financial gain. The incentives came from a capitated payment system under which Gaines was contracted by the insurance company, MetLife.[14]

The lawsuit charged that Dr. Gaines failed to detect Ching's cancer at an early stage because of his reluctance to order expensive tests due to his financial arrangements with MetLife. During the three months when Ching sought treatment for persistent abdominal bleeding and pelvic pain, the suit alleged, Dr. Gaines kept turning down her request that he refer her to a specialist.[15]

The suit alleged that in an early visit to his office in August 1992, Gaines ordered one ultrasound test, at a cost of $225, which failed to adequately explain a palpable mass. The plaintiffs claimed that since the cost of the procedure was equal to roughly eight months of Ching's monthly $27.94 capitation fee, the doctor had already lost money on her, which could have made him hesitant to order more tests. According to the plaintiffs, this resulted in a late diagnosis and therefore in Ching's death.

Before the case was heard during the fall of 1995, legal experts believed that it would be the first in the state of California that would directly challenge the use of HMO payment systems because of their effect on physician behavior. However, the trial judge reduced the case to one of simple malpractice against the doctor for failing to properly diagnose Ching's condition.[16] Furthermore, since MetLife was not even named as a defendant, the use of capitation arrangements was never directly challenged.[17] While the case failed in its mission of successfully challenging the use of these types of incentives, it served to powerfully highlight the tensions inherent in prepaid health care.

Recent headlines have also raised suspicions about other organizational policies that may direct doctors away from serving the best interests of their patients. Most noteworthy is the use of "gag orders" in contracts with physicians. Allegedly, these "disparagement clauses" prohibit the disclosure of financial incentives, treatment options not covered by patient policies, and remarks that can be interpreted as "undermining the confidence of enrollees" in the health plan.[18] Various accounts report that physicians have been disciplined or have had their contracts terminated for communications that could be interpreted as disparaging to the contracting organization.[19] In some extreme cases, physicians have been prohibited from informing their patients that they were seeking a specialty referral until such a referral had been approved by the organization.[20]

Accompanying these potential ethical conflicts for individual physicians, are ones which directly involve the *organization*. Concerns have also been raised about various *organizational*-level cost-saving practices which may result in significant harm to patients. These potential conflicts were manifested in two recent cases, which also received a great amount of publicity.

The first case involved the controversial policy of various organizations, most notably Kaiser, which established that mothers of newborns normally must be discharged from the hospital within twenty-four hours of delivery. Critics, who have labeled the practice "drive-through deliveries," claim that the policy was a morally unjustifiable intrusion on the patient-physician relationship. The practice, they state, amounts to a third party, like Kaiser, rather than a physician, making decisions regarding when to release patients. Also important is the fact that the period in question represents a much shorter time frame than what had been customary, prompting fear that the health of both the mother and child was jeopardized.[21] The case became such a focal point of controversy that it provided the impetus for several state legislatures to pass laws that would force insurers to pay for 48-hour stays for normal births and 96-hour stays for Cesarean section births.[22] In the aftermath, legislation with similar requirements was also signed into law at the federal level.[23]

The second case, which was the subject of a much discussed *Time* magazine cover story, involved questions over the interpretation of clauses in managed care contracts which exclude procedures because of their "experimental" nature. The case also illustrated the debate over whether or not appeals over such denials and other utilization review decisions should be decided by an independent party.[24]

The particular situation involved a Health Net enrollee, thirty-four-year-old Christy deMeurers, who was diagnosed with breast cancer and later died of the disease. Despite the recommendations of her doctors, Health Net denied an expensive bone marrow transplant on the grounds that it was "experimental or investigative," although the organization had earlier approved the procedure for at least one other patient. After a series of appeals and visits to other doctors, the deMeurers family finally sued Health Net in 1993 to force the insurer to cover the cost of the procedure, which it refused to do. DeMeurers eventually underwent the procedure after officials at the UCLA medical center determined that their institution would pay for it. She died in March 1995, only a year and a half after receiving the treatment.

The case was eventually heard in arbitration in October 1995. The panel found against Health Net on several counts and awarded the deMeurers family a million-dollar judgment. The arbitrators ruled that the procedure was not experimental, since it was increasingly being used with some success as a cancer treatment. The arbitrators also ruled that the term "investigative" was too ambiguous to stand as the basis for denial of treatment.[25] Following the case, Health Net changed its procedures for handling appeals for bone marrow transplants in non-standard cases and now sends them to an independent review organization.[26] Health Net revamped its policies for experimental treatments, but similar cases involving other managed care organizations continue to make headlines.

PROFITS VS. PATIENTS

Each of these cases has contributed to a heightened level of public discourse concerning the morality of managed care practices. To many critics, any pressure on physicians to curb treatments infringes upon medicine's long-held moral norms that uphold the primacy of patient well-being. They argue that when physicians work for managed care organizations through "staff model" HMOs, or are under contract to them through Independent Practice Associations (IPAs) or variations thereof, their loyalties are torn from the Hippocratic Oath's moral norm of serving as the patient's advocate. Adding financial incentives and "gag orders" to physician contracts and the related profit motive of corporations into the equation only further divides physician loyalties. Doctors become what Edmund Pellegrino has termed "double or triple agents," who must balance patient needs, their own economic well-being, and financial returns to shareholders.[27]

Critics have raised concerns over harm to the broader society as well as to individual patients. In particular, they question whether the pursuit of profit by corporations in the industry will lead them to exclusively engage in health care practices that contribute to their bottom line.[28] For example, some fear that managed care organizations will act like traditional insurers, who maximize profits through selectively offering policies only to healthier members of the population.[29] There is a hidden incentive to "cherry pick" by attracting only the healthiest subscribers and by ignoring populations that are expensive to treat.[30] Consequently, overall community health will suffer.

Accusations also have been levied against managed care organizations for unsavory marketing techniques, such as persuasive advertising which borders on deceit and outright fraud, in order to sign up Medicare beneficiaries.[31] In some arrangements, salespersons have received commissions per person enrolled, prompting concern that greed will lead to the consideration of the salesperson's best interest rather than the patient's, in the enrollment of new subscribers.[32]

Some observers have also raised the concern that profit-seeking organizations "skim the economic cream" out of the health care system. In the past, the practice of "cost-shifting" was used to pay for indigent care. Patients who could pay were charged higher rates in order to cover the costs of those who could not. Managed care plans eliminate this source of financing because of their lower reimbursement rates. In effect, for-profit plans extract these savings as profits, leaving fewer resources to "shift." Moreover, if capitation payment arrangements grow concomitantly with enrollment in managed care organizations, the practice of cost-shifting will further diminish. Physicians and hospitals will find it much more difficult to provide care for the poor, since they will receive a set amount for paying patients regardless of the actual amount of services rendered, leaving less to cover indigent care.[33]

In addition to these controversies, profit-seeking managed care organizations have also been accused of bringing some of the more deplorable aspects of corporate behavior and free-market competition into medicine. For instance, some critics have noted that HMOs implementing potentially harmful cost-savings mechanisms were simultaneously pursuing large-scale mergers and acquisitions, at the cost of millions of dollars. For example, the *failed* merger between Health Systems International, the corporate parent of Health Net, and WellPoint Health Networks cost approximately $20 million in payments to lawyers, investment bankers, and other expenses.[34] Many of these organizations also pay multimillion dollar salaries to their top executives. These practices have prompted a vocal public protest that such frivolous spending and individual enrichment should not occur at the expense of the ill health of others, especially when some treatments are even being withheld in the name of fiscal responsibility.

MEDICINE AND THE MARKETPLACE: AN UNEASY TENSION

These issues have led many to conclude that business and medicine should remain in mutually exclusive domains because of their diametrically opposed moral paradigms. Simply put, the traditional "good" for business has been and continues to be profit, while the "good" for medicine is the well-being of patients. As a result, these organizations cannot simultaneously serve their business interests without defaulting upon their obligations as health care providers. In terms similar to those of Bristow, Wendy Mariner holds that:

> Those who argue that MCO's should operate like efficient businesses in a competitive marketplace are, in effect, arguing for no standards at all. A free-market approach stresses organizing and delivering health care in an economically efficient, value-free way. This effectively precludes the imposition of normative values on MCO's.[35]

Such concerns are widely held and warrant our attention. However, there are also many vocal supporters of managed care who focus on the positive contributions of this emerging form of medical delivery. In particular, they point out that within our climate of spiraling health care costs and fiscal scarcity, market-based incentives must be utilized in order to control medical expenditures and to keep health insurance affordable. Since society lacks a limitless pool of financial resources to cover all of its medical demands, physicians and third parties must be involved in the cost-control process.

Under traditional fee-for-service reimbursement arrangements, patients are presumed to be "cost-unconscious consumers" who expect unlimited quantities of procedures with little concern for expense and/or effectiveness. Their "unconsciousness" stems from the fact that third-party payers, namely employers and insurers, have typically covered the true costs of care. Moreover, it is clearly in the financial interests of physicians to prescribe unlimited procedures, since they are reimbursed for each service.[36] These factors have contributed to exploding health care costs and have heightened accessibility issues, placing health care out of the reach of the most unfortunate members of society. E. Haavi Morreim states that demands for "everything available" violate broader norms of justice by jeopardizing the availability of health care resources for the "many" in favor of the claims of the few.[37] Supporters of managed care claim that, in effect, managed care reverses the older incentive system and instead encourages consciousness of costs and limits on wasteful care.

In their response to situations in which patients may be harmed by cost-cutting incentives, as in the case of Joyce Ching, spokespersons for managed care organizations argue that it is the responsibility of the primary care physicians, who act as gatekeepers to uphold their patients' best interests. They assert that payment methods such as capitation are useful tools to encourage physicians to be more cost-conscious and to perform procedures or make referrals only when they are truly necessary. Furthermore, they claim that in most cases in which they are used, capitation payments are fairly calculated and are designed to cover the costs of health care without forcing the doctor into a dilemma. Thus, in these cases it is the responsibility of individual physicians to retain the ethical standards of their profession.[38]

Spokespersons for the managed care industry also argue that the widespread concerns over profit-seeking behavior which damages patient care are unwarranted. Despite the few well-publicized cases, they claim that cost-containment has no noticeable negative effect on quality, since on the whole, only wasteful treatments are eliminated.[39] These advocates argue that a health care system subject to market discipline, functioning like other businesses, will necessarily hold costs down while improving quality.[40] In addition to seeking to avoid malpractice suits, a health care organization must behave just like any other business that wants to survive in the long run, by acting in a manner that pleases its customers. Susan Pisano, a spokesperson for the Group Health Association of America (the leading trade association for HMOs), states that managed care is

> the only system with every incentive to keep people healthy, whether that means we prevent disease in the first place, treat problems early or take charge of the management of chronic disease. People who function poorly cost more to the health plan and to society.[41]

Kaiser officials employed a similar line of reasoning in their response to allegations that their early release policy would harm mothers and newborns. Kaiser representatives stated that it would make no sense to release patients before they were ready, since such a practice will ultimately cost the organization more in the long run if mothers or infants must return for treatment.[42]

Even some of the critics of the more controversial practices of managed care organizations acknowledge their contributions. For example, Jerome Kassirer, editor of *The New England Journal of Medicine*, notes:

> Patients stay in the hospital for fewer days, many surgical procedures that previously required hospitalization are now safely performed in day surgery, there is far more attention to preventative care, many medical practices have been standardized to produce better outcomes, and satisfying patients has become an explicit goal.[43]

Despite the fact that there is some level of agreement about positive contributions of managed care, many are skeptical of the mo-

rality of managed care as a whole. David Thomasma has stated that the purpose of any health reform plan must be to improve quality of care for individual patients, while simultaneously reducing the economic burdens on the populace and on government third-party payers.[44] Currently, there is intense debate over whether or not managed care, especially when for-profit organizations are involved in its delivery, is able to achieve both goals. While advocates of managed care claim that these organizations can meet both objectives, well-publicized cases seem to provide evidence that financial goals can only be achieved at the direct expense of patient well-being.

THE CURRENT LEGAL ENVIRONMENT

In response to the current levels of public concern, legislatures have been busily considering a host of proposed measures to regulate the activities of managed care organizations. It is becoming quite clear that the law is failing to keep pace with the rapid changes in the health care system. However, there is vast disagreement over the extent to which legal measures can or should be used to restrain some of the practices of managed care.

Nevertheless, numerous legal measures, in addition to those prohibiting "drive-through deliveries," have recently been implemented or are in the process of being considered. President Clinton has also proposed a federal-level patient "bill of rights" to safeguard the interests of patients. The newest proposed legislation would provide information about quality of care, allow patients to have coverage for the nearest hospital in an emergency, and guarantee access to specialists. In addition, a system for appealing denied treatments would be put into place. Many of the laws being contemplated are similar in scope to the AMA-supported Patient Protection Act, which failed to pass into law when it was introduced in Congress in 1994. If the measure had gained enough support for enactment, it would have required the Secretary of Health and Human Services to establish federal standards for the certification of managed care plans. Insurance plans would have been required to disclose the criteria they use to select and exclude physicians from their networks, to give doctors the right to appeal their exclusion from a contracted panel, and to furnish doctors with a reason for dismissal.[45] The proposed legislation would have offered consumers various protections, including standards for utilization review, full disclosure about financial arrangements within their plans, prevention of discrimination based upon pre-existing conditions, and a required point-of-service option that would allow visits to doctors outside of the plan for higher fees.[46]

While such measures have yet to be established on a federal level, several states have enacted all or parts of the key provisions of the Patient Protection Act during the past two years, with the support of state medical associations and various consumer groups. In California, the state in which managed care has made the greatest inroads, several such bills have been signed into law. They include measures which establish minimum requirements for utilization reviewers, protect physicians who fight a denied utilization review decision on behalf of a patient against retaliation from the managed care plan, and require plans to establish grievance systems and complaint hot lines.[47] As a result of cases such as the one involving deMeurers and Health Net, a bill was signed into law to offer further protection to patients with terminal illnesses. The legislation will give these patients the right to have their cases reviewed by an independent panel of doctors if they are denied "experimental" treatments.[48]

Several other states have enacted bills which allow direct access to specific specialists without "gatekeeper" approval, establish "any willing provider" provisions under which any physician who meets basic requirements can join a network, and outlaw "gag orders" by mandating information disclosure to patients about treatment options.[49] In some states, voters are being asked to consider ballot initiatives that would attempt to curb some of these controversial practices.[50]

In addition to the work of legislatures and the initiative process, a body of case law[51] is emerging, albeit slowly and in a rather disjointed fashion. To date, courts have established that managed care organizations can be held liable for their activities under various legal theories. First, managed care organizations, like hospitals, can be held directly responsible under malpractice laws for negligent actions which harm patients. Second, in some cases they can be held vicariously liable for the actions of physicians who are under contract to them through the agency doctrine of *respondeat superior*, provided these doctors have been "held out" as employees.[52] Third, courts have established that faulty cost-control mechanisms such as utilization review procedures at variance with medical norms can be a cause for liability.[53] Similarly, managed care organizations have also found themselves accountable for bad faith denial of claims, the most common basis for the extension of liability.[54]

Despite these developments, however, the overall legal environment has not kept pace with the rapid changes in health care. Legislators have been placed in the unenviable position of trying to develop policies that meet societal demands for the dual goals of limitless treatments and improved economic accessibility. Within the constraints of current resource limits, these aims necessarily conflict. Thus, elected officials are at odds over how best to encourage enrollment in managed care organizations because of their fiscal promise, while at the same time protecting patients and physicians in a manner which will not negate the cost-savings achieved. As a result, many of the most controversial aspects of managed care are not addressed through legislation, leaving patients and physicians in precarious positions. Laws governing the most controversial financial incentives to reduce health care expenditures, such as capitation payment systems, risk sharing, and bonus pools arrangements have been slow to develop. Moreover, there are no uniform federal regulations establishing minimum qualifications for utilization reviewers, or federal mandates which require disclosure to patients of financial incentives given to physicians or of the availability of non-covered treatment options.

The various measures mentioned earlier clearly offer some level of increased protection to patients and physicians. However, the absence of federal standards leaves the legal guidelines which surround managed care with great variations from state to state. Moreover, state measures are often preempted by Federal Employment Retirement Income Security Act (ERISA) laws, which were established in 1974 to protect employer retirement plans from lawsuits that could threaten their financial integrity. A 1987 court decision ruled that health benefits provided under an employer-sponsored plan are also under the jurisdiction of ERISA, protecting employers' rights to hold down costs and to preserve their ability to offer plans to their employees. In effect, this denies the right of patients to seek legal recourse against the employer and the employer's plan under state measures, even in cases of wrongful death caused by a faulty denial of benefit.[55] Several other courts have reached similar rulings in ERISA-related cases. One ruling expressed concern that such a preemption could lead to cost-free errors on the part of managed care organizations.[56] As a result of the ERISA preemption, physicians are often the sole entities legally accountable for decisions that result in harm to patients.[57]

Many of the most promising legal cases which would have addressed some of the newer and most controversial practices, and which could have set important precedents, have been reduced in scope or settled out of court. These developments have further slowed the evolution of case law. Although several courts have stated that immunity is not granted to third-party payers for practices that bring harm to patients just because public policy favors cost-containment, the extent of legal liability is still unclear.[58] For instance, no resolution has been attained in several cases which have focused on whether the managed care organization itself could be held liable for patient harm through decisions that were altered by financial incentives, such as capitation and controlled access through gatekeeping. As noted earlier, the case involving Joyce Ching and MetLife failed in its mission of mounting a direct legal challenge to the use of capitation arrangements, despite the promise of landmark status. Another case, in which an MCO was sued because its capitation payment system allegedly resulted in a physician withholding a referral from a cancer patient, was settled prior to trial.[59] A more recent case which challenged the role of gatekeepers ended up focusing exclusively on the role of the gatekeeping physician, because the ERISA preemption was determined to preclude the naming of the MCO in the suit.[60]

In addition to a shortage of cases dealing with payment systems, there is also a dearth of established precedence with respect to interpretations of the meaning of the term "experimental," when treatments are denied under its auspices. The family of Christy deMeurers was awarded a million-dollar judgment against

Health Net for the insurer's narrow interpretation of the clause and its heavy-handed interference with the patient-physician relationship, but the case was heard in arbitration and therefore is not binding as precedent in any court of law. In another case involving Health Net, the family of cancer victim Nelene Fox was awarded a $90 million judgment by a jury for a similar denial of an autologous bone marrow transplant.[61] The jury's verdict was based in part on the fact that Health Net had previously approved the procedure for two other women.[62] What remains unclear, however, are situations in which no appeal for a particular procedure within a plan has been previously approved for another patient because the term "experimental" has been consistently, but falsely, applied in utilization decisions.

Underlying the disagreements in the formation of law is a contentious ethical debate over the extent to which public policy *should* govern the activities of managed care organizations. In general, supporters of various legislative proposals and initiatives, including spokespersons representing organized medicine, wish to see more curbs written into law in order to protect individual patients and physicians from the growing power of managed care organizations.

In contrast, some supporters of managed care would like to see fewer restrictions. They argue that increased aggregate-level costs are a direct consequence of unnecessary legislative interference. One industry spokesperson points out that a cataract operation which used to require a one- to two-week hospital stay, and is now performed as an outpatient procedure, is indicative of the fact that the law cannot keep pace with cost savings achieved through new technology.[63] Reactionary legislation such as mandating minimum stays for mothers of newborns, in which patient health is not in jeopardy, can similarly limit the medical gains and subsequent cost savings made possible by technological advances. As a result of such legislation, they argue, other patients are hurt because limited resources are allocated that could be used elsewhere in the health care system.

More radically, a few observers have suggested that physicians operating in managed care organizations be held to a different standard of care than fee-for-service doctors, in recognition of cost-control goals.[64] In particular, physicians should be legally freed from the individual patient-centered fiduciary responsibilities of the older model in the name of justice to other policyholders in the plan, who may suffer if a few individuals consume too many plan resources.[65] These commentators have interpreted several recent legal decisions as giving providers some leeway to practice a more conservative, cost-efficient style of medicine.[66]

These disagreements and the sheer volume of proposed legal changes that legislators, jurists, and voters are all being asked to consider present vexing challenges. It is imperative that the underlying ethical conflicts over the role of managed care and particularly of for-profit organizations be discussed and resolved before more policies are implemented. Otherwise, we run the risk of enacting measures in the name of reform which neither protect patients and physicians, nor achieve the goal of cost-containment and improved access to care.

Two Reframing the Debate

Perspectives Critical of Managed Care

The moral challenges prompted by managed care seem to offer a simple choice between the profit-seeking behavior of modern corporations and the healing mission of medicine, as practiced under the traditional fee-for-service model. As noted in the introduction, much of the current literature presents the debate under a simple rubric with only two perspectives: arguments against managed care and arguments in support of it.[1] Given the overlap in the arguments of the respective critics and supporters of managed care, a simple dichotomy is helpful in terms of a broad overview of the issues. But this greatly obscures the complexity of the debate. There are multiple perspectives, each with its own set of assumptions and values, from which arguments are being advanced. Placing all of the proponents of managed care in one category and all their adversaries in the other obscures the fact that within these two categories are strongly conflicting opinions about the norms which should guide health care delivery. In addition, as I noted earlier, such a portrayal encourages purely destructive forms of criticism. One can advance arguments against managed care without ever articulating a positive description of an alternative; similarly, one can criticize "traditional" health care without ever addressing the moral issues of managed care.

This chapter and the next set the stage for a deeper evaluation of the moral viability of for-profit organizations in managed care. The standard two-part rubric will be broadened to include commonly omitted perspectives, which either offer reform alternatives to managed care, or support for particular variations of it. Two benefits accrue from such an expanded view. First, we will see that none of the perspectives from which criticisms are being advanced against managed care are free from shortcomings of their own, and hence, the solution to ethical dilemmas in health care delivery is not as simple as the abolition of the emerging model. Second, we will find that there are many supporters of this newer model of health care who are not champions of *laissez-faire* medicine, contrary to what many critics believe. Indeed, many advocates of managed care are wary of some of the ways it is currently being implemented.

THE MORAL TYPOLOGY

In place of the common dichotomy, the moral debate surrounding managed care can be represented by a typology with six different perspectives. Of the six types, three support managed care and three reject it. However, these perspectives can be further and more accurately distinguished by their views of two factors, which can be placed along two continuums. These relationships are represented graphically in the following diagram:

DIAGRAM 1
Typology of the Ethical Perspectives on Health Care Delivery

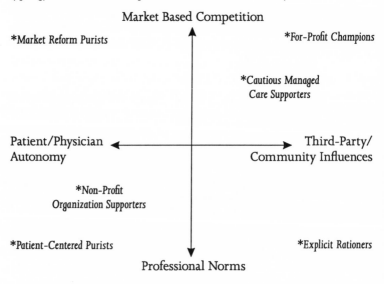

The two continuums in Diagram 1 form four quadrants into which each of these perspectives can be placed. The horizontal axis is a continuum representing beliefs about the degree to which medical care should be "managed" by influences external to the patient-physician relationship.[2] This represents one of the major points of division in competing visions of health care delivery. At one end of the continuum is the view that individual patients, in conjunction with their physicians and apart from any other considerations, should be the final arbiters of prescribed health care procedures. This perspective values individual autonomy, one of the traditional precepts of medical ethics, in health care decisions. At the other end of the continuum is the view that since many medical procedures are wasteful, care must be "managed." Fiscal conservation becomes a significant aspect of medical practice. The moral concern from this perspective is that an exclusive focus on individual wants violates egalitarian conceptions of distributive and intergenerational justice, since there are limited aggregate health care resources.

The second continuum, represented by the vertical axis, distinguishes perspectives according to their beliefs about the basis of accountability for cost and quality in the health care system. Since all of these voices at least ostensibly acknowledge growing social concerns about rising health care costs and the maintenance of quality, they can be distinguished with respect to the guarantor for these factors. On one end of the continuum are those who believe that market-based competition, especially the profit motive, is the best vehicle to ensure cost-efficient quality medicine. Morally speaking, adherents of this viewpoint distrust the older model of medicine in which patients had few incentives to monitor costs and efficiency. They believe it facilitated professional dominance by physicians, artificially escalated prices, and aided in the proliferation of incentives for waste. On the other end of the continuum are those who reject market-based competition and argue that either the exclusive use of professional medical norms, or community-chosen priorities in conjunction with such norms, are the best means to assure that aggregate health care spending is reduced.

Using these two continuums, each of the six types of moral perspectives that will be developed here fall into one of four quadrants, located at different points on each continuum. As this typology illustrates, the moral debate over managed care and the participation of for-profit organizations within it is much broader and more complex than it appears. Diagram 2 summarizes the positions of each of these perspectives on managed care and the role of the profit motive within it.

DIAGRAM 2
Views on Managed Care and the Profit Motive

Type	Managed Care	Profit
1. Patient-Centered Purists	Reject	Reject
2. Market Reform Purists (MSAs)	Reject	Support*
3. Explicit Rationers	Reject	Reject
4. Cautious Managed Care Supporters	Tenuous Support	Tenuous Support
5. For-Profit Managed Care Champions	Support	Support
6. Non-Profit Organization Supporters	Support	Reject

*Advocates of Medical Savings Accounts tend to reject competition among managed care organizations and instead support competition among individual physicians.

These perspectives are placed in their respective positions in the typology because of their stance with respect to the moral viability of managed care as a medical delivery option. The rest of this chapter and the next describe in detail the moral arguments and preferred policies advanced by each of the "types," beginning with those which are critical of managed care.

PATIENT-CENTERED PURISTS

As the name "Patient-Centered Purists" suggests, adherents to this perspective are critical of managed care for its departure from the traditional ethical norms of medicine, which place primacy on the well-being of individual patients regardless of financial considerations. They fear that with the current changes in health care delivery, the sacred trust between doctor and patient will be largely abolished, except for the fortunate few who can still afford more expensive fee-for-service reimbursement insurance policies.[3]

It is important to note that many in this category do not explicitly state that they wish to return to fee-for-service arrangements. Some voice purely destructive forms of criticism. However, judging by their stated concerns that the influence of third parties and market competition on health care will lead doctors to abandon their role as patient-centered advocates, and their lack of an explicitly stated alternative, one can surmise that they indeed favor the preservation of the fee-for-service system.[4] Though it remains uncertain how many individual physicians actually support this perspective, much of the rhetoric that has traditionally come from organized medicine falls into this category.[5]

Patient-Centered Purists advocate a return to an older model of medicine, under which third-party influences on care decisions would be minimized and professional norms, rather than impersonal market forces, would ensure moral accountability in the practice of medicine. In particular, they argue that conventional fee-for-service arrangements are the best means to ensure that physicians will act in a manner that honors the traditional moral standards of medicine. As a result, they can be placed in the lower-left quadrant of the typology presented earlier.

Some Patient-Centered Purists acknowledge that fee-for-service arrangements are not free from conflicts of interest, since there are built-in incentives for physicians to overprescribe in order to maximize their financial gain. However, they argue that in this model, the best interests of the physician and the patient are most closely aligned. In addition, they argue, individual physicians are free to resolve ethical dilemmas in the patient's interest under fee-for-service arrangements. In contrast, under managed care arrangements, conflicts of interest are worse because the costs of favoring the patient's interests are much greater to the physician.[6] Since doctors are employed directly by managed care organizations or medical groups under contract to them, physicians who practice with their patients' best interests in mind can be dismissed from provider panels for a lack of compliance with financial goals. Doctors, they argue, are under immense pressure from their employers to cut costs and perhaps corners.[7] Thus, doctors are less at liberty under the newer arrangements to favor their patients' interests.

Because of their interest in the well-being of individual patients, Patient-Centered Purists cite several *paradigmatic* concerns about the ethics behind the very concepts and ideals of managed care. First, regardless of the profit-status of organizations involved in its delivery, they argue that managed care is, at its heart, a rationing scheme, since it limits care for individual patients for the sake of preserving resources for others. In particular, they charge that cost-cutting mechanisms such as restricted access to doctors and limits on the use of expensive procedures are really forms of rationing disguised under other names.[8] Doctors who are paid through capitation arrangements are faced with bedside rationing decisions, since patients are competing for care provided with limited dollars. This places physicians in the tenuous position of choosing between the well-being of some patients versus others. Consequently, capitation arrangements violate a long-held norm of medicine that once physicians enter a relationship with a patient, the individual patient's best interests must be the sole consideration in decision making.[9]

Second, they fear that the entry of large-scale organizations into medical delivery, especially profit-seeking ones, will irreparably damage medicine. Patient-Centered Purists are particularly concerned that organizations governed by a business ethic rather than the traditional medical ethic will damage the moral norms of physicians and will make profit a primary consideration in medical decisions.[10]

The quote cited from AMA president Bristow in the introduction is representative of these paradigmatic concerns about the collision of the business ethic with the medical ethic. The goal of business, it is assumed, is to increase shareholder wealth, while the aim of medicine is to cure patients without regard for financial considerations. One physician captures the spirit of beliefs about these differences by stating that unlike doctors, "insurance company executives take no oath whatsoever, and their 'morality' is purely profit driven."[11]

Echoing these concerns, several commentators have pointed

to some of the metaphors that have developed since managed care has grown to its present state as indicative of the lengths to which medicine is moving away from the patient-centered ethic and focusing on the bottom line. Edmund Pellegrino has noted that the honorable title of "physician" has been replaced by "case manager," "fund holder," and "gatekeeper." These replacements, he fears, will lead doctors away from their traditional commitments and into an ethical framework in which their behavior will be guided by the principle of *caveat emptor*.[12] Along similar lines, Jerome Kassirer has commented that for some MCOs, patient care is viewed as a *cost* of being in the "health care business." He cites the term "medical-loss ratio," which is used to describe the resources actually spent on health care, as evidence of the increasing encroachment of corporate conglomerates on the medical profession.[13] Other critics have also noted the irony of the use of marketing-oriented nomenclature, such as naming an organization "Maxicare," "when the obvious incentives of such organizations are to restrain rather than maximize the use of medical services."[14]

Based upon these paradigmatic concerns, Patient-Centered Purists cite some *specific* shortcomings which they believe will harm patients, physicians, and society in general as managed care replaces traditional fee-for-service medicine. They allege that on the level of patient-physician relationships, financial incentives undermine the doctor's commitment to be the patient's advocate. The case involving Joyce Ching (chapter 1) is an apparent example. Physicians will be tempted either to not prescribe needed procedures or to resist making a referral to a specialist who is better trained to treat the condition in question.

A further concern is that other cost-savings mechanisms of managed care organizations will greatly damage the quality of care that patients receive, again due to the intrusion of third parties into the patient-physician relationship.[15] For example, prospective utilization reviews by either personnel of the managed care organizations or independent utilization review organizations hired by an MCO can overturn the recommendations of a patient's doctor, though there is little data to indicate the frequency with which this occurs. This can result in the denial of various types of care, including treatment by specialists and the use of expensive procedures.

In addition, observers raise the specter of the temptation to withhold treatments that are costly to implement regardless of therapeutic value, including expensive emergency care.[16] An apparent example is the situation in which Christy deMeurers was denied an experimental treatment for cancer. Some observers worry that the criteria of "medical necessity" or "appropriateness" used by reviewers to approve expensive procedures are inadequately determined and could place quality and thus patient health in jeopardy. Critics also fear that faceless bureaucrats in far-away offices, many of whom are professional administrators rather than physicians, are engaging in the practice of medicine through control of reimbursement decisions.

Managed care is accused of abridging what is considered to be an "ideal" patient-physician relationship in several other ways. To many observers, a long-term relationship of trust between patient and physician has actual therapeutic value. An ongoing affiliation can lead to the recognition of diagnostic patterns and histories in a patient that medical records cannot adequately communicate. Such a relationship also engenders trust in confidentiality, leading to more accurate diagnosis and efficient treatment decisions. However, these associations are threatened. Many employers offer only one plan with limited provider panels, severely undermining the ability of patients to choose their own physicians.[17] Some employers also frequently switch to cheaper plans, sometimes on a yearly basis. As a result, many patients lack the continuity considered to be critical in the ideal patient-physician relationship.[18] High disenrollment figures are cited in order to highlight this problem. For instance, Ezekial Emanuel and Allen Brett report that HMOs indicate that approximately 10 to 15 percent, and up to 30 percent, of subscribers disenroll each year.[19] Moreover, as many as 40 percent of new enrollees in some surveys reported that they had to change doctors when they enrolled in their plan.[20] These critics further allege that once patients are in an actual relationship with a physician, the long-held doctrine of "informed consent" is impinged upon by the "gag orders" mentioned in the previous chapter.

Patient-Centered Purists are highly skeptical that managed care can achieve its cost-savings goals without damaging society in significant ways. They respond to spokespersons for MCOs, who claim that only wasteful procedures are being withheld, by arguing that the measurements of quality and hence "waste" that are used to make such judgments are faulty and underdeveloped. Several commentators dismiss high patient satisfaction rates reported by managed care plans as inadequate indices of "quality," because the plans' surveys rely on visible amenities rather than educated judgments about medical care.[21] They claim that lower premium costs are the direct result not of improvements in efficiency, but of reduced benefits and limiting choices of providers, both of which are damaging to patients.[22]

Given these many concerns, Patient-Centered Purists would like to see a return to fee-for-service medicine. They would rather rely on the professional ethics of individual physicians than on the marketplace to encourage and monitor the practice of cost-efficient medicine. Although the official statement from the American Medical Association's Council on Ethical and Judicial Affairs does not condemn managed care outright, many groups in organized medicine have sought to limit the power of managed care organizations and to restore fee-for-service arrangements through the legislative process.[23]

Various proposals have contained elements that would weaken the ability of managed care organizations to use their various cost-cutting mechanisms. In particular, some groups have sought to dismantle the use of selective contracting through the introduction of "any willing provider" provisions in reform legislation.[24] Furthermore, in a surprise to most observers, some professional medical associations have gone against long-held disavowals of "socialized medicine" and have actually endorsed single-payer (vs. employer-based) proposals, believing that this financing method offers the best chance to preserve the dominance of fee-for-service arrangements.[25]

MARKET REFORM PURISTS

In addition to Patient-Centered Purists, a growing number of other voices seek to restore the dominance of fee-for-service arrangements. "Market Reform Purists" express similar moral concerns about the interference of third parties in the patient-physician relationship.[26] They are also concerned about the "portability" problem when employees lose or change jobs.[27] However, unlike Patient-Centered Purists, Market Reform Purists believe that financial matters should be a primary consideration in the practice of medicine. Furthermore, they contend that the market is the best basis to ensure cost consciousness and the monitoring of quality.

Market Reform Purists express serious concerns about rising aggregate-level health care costs. Consequently, they are highly critical of the older fee-for-service model in which there were no incentives for cost-efficiency, since insurance claims were reimbursed with little regard for the expense, degree of medical necessity, or actual benefit of the care rendered. In effect, this shielded patients and physicians from the real cost of care. As a result, these purists do not trust the exclusive use of professional medical norms to guarantee fiscal accountability. These views place Market Reform Purists on the left side of Diagram 1, but on the opposite end of the accountability continuum from Patient-Centered Purists.

Market Reform Purists argue that an effective model of health care reform must not proceed on the assumption that patients are ignorant and unable to exercise intelligent market discipline.[28] Thus, they support free-market reforms as the most efficient means of health care delivery. However, instead of advocating competition and price reductions occurring at the level of third parties such as managed care organizations, they argue that patients should be given direct incentives to reduce the use of wasteful procedures and to find lower-cost providers. These commentators predict that this will achieve the societal goal of lower aggregate costs.

Given these beliefs, it is accurate to state that Market Reform Purists, rather than adherents of other perspectives supporting managed care in the name of "free-market reform," are the true "free-marketers" in this debate. In fact, Market Reform Purists reject the current system of managed care partially because it does not go far enough in terms of market-based reforms. They note that the actual "end consumers," the patients, are separated from the actual purchase of health care insurance. Although adherents of this perspective acknowledge that incentive for waste was more acute in the older fee-for-service model, they claim that a similar problem exists under managed care. Since patients still do not directly feel the actual effects of prescribed care in their own pocketbooks, there are no disincentives to demand every available option for treatment. Because of these factors, Market Reform Purists note that the health care system is not subject to the price mechanism of true market discipline. From their perspective, the emerging managed care system that is being ballyhooed as "free-market" is really an "anti-market system masquerading as capitalistic and market oriented."[29] In effect, they contend that this has further contributed to our fiscal crisis, since many patients still regard health care as a "free" good, "because someone else is paying for the care."[30]

To support their case, Market Reform Purists cite various studies indicating that financial incentives directly reduce the use of care. One set of studies often mentioned is a series conducted by the Rand Corporation, which concluded that families with lower co-payments spent a significant amount more on health care with no noticeable improvement in health outcomes than those who had higher payments.[31] These studies also suggested that moving from "free" care to a fee-for-service plan with a 25 percent copayment could reduce total outlays by 23 percent.[32] Thus, Market Reform Purists conclude that policies that make consumers more cognizant of expenditures are promising in terms of reaching the goal of lower aggregate costs.

Market Reform Purists note that the ability of consumers to "vote with their dollars" and exercise market discipline is marginal, since for most, the selection of plans is limited to those offered by employers. This factor artificially weakens the forces of supply and demand, leading to higher prices and decreased efficiency. As such, the current managed care system further erodes the traditional consumer role of watchdog as it exists in the market for other goods and services.[33]

All of these factors have led Market Reform Purists to conclude that a system in which true market forces and values are the means of reform has not really been tried at all. They believe that a system in which health care providers are forced to directly market their product to the consumer, and not to his or her employer, would be the most efficient since reform based upon a pure market mechanism would then be utilized.[34]

Proponents of this perspective contend that medical delivery would work best with a fee-for-service method under which individual patients negotiate prices directly with their own choice of provider plans, doctors, clinics, and hospitals.[35] As a policy measure, they argue this would be best accomplished through the use of Medical Savings Accounts, otherwise known as "Medical IRAs," which would serve to create greater market pressure by encouraging consumer responsibility and cost consciousness.[36]

Medical Savings Accounts work in a manner much like proposed school voucher systems. Instead of contracting with insurers such as MCOs, health care payers such as private employers or the government would place a yearly sum into an account that a patient would draw upon for routine low-cost medical expenses. Any amount left at the end of the year can either be kept by the patient as "income" or rolled over into the account and added to the next year's contribution. Funds not spent during the person's years of employment could be used to pay for retirement health care costs or rolled over into a pension fund.[37] True "insurance" would be reserved for high-cost medical situations in which the cost of care exceeds the total in the expense account. In order for this plan to work most efficiently, the current tax code would have to be reformed. Market Reform Purists argue that under the present system, a tremendous incentive for waste is created because out-of-pocket payments are not tax-deductible, while 100 percent of the benefit received from employer contributions to insurance plans can be written off. Thus, most employers would rather enroll their employees in extremely expensive low-deductible insurance plans, which create incentives for waste since patients bear little of the true cost of care. Market Reform Purists contend that a great deal of savings could be realized if less expensive, high-deductible plans were purchased and the savings placed, tax free, into MSAs to meet low cost, out-of-pocket expenses.[38]

In a typical MSA arrangement, the employer would place an

amount of around $2,000 or $3,000 into an account for an employee and his or her family to cover out-of-pocket expenses. Though the evidence is limited, it has been estimated that as of 1993, less than 12.5 percent of patients had claims in excess of $2,000 in a given year.[39] Thus, most employees would be able to meet their medical expenditures with the amount set aside. The employer or another purchaser would also buy a high-deductible indemnity plan for the employee and his or her family to cover catastrophic illnesses. While estimates vary by geographic region and other factors, the typical cost of purchasing a high-deductible policy in conjunction with the amount placed into the Medical Savings Account would roughly equal the amount now being spent per year by employers on health policies for the same family.[40] Although employers would pay roughly the equivalent of what they have been paying for traditional policies, the real benefit to them is that their costs would not rise in the long term, because the actual users of health care will have the incentives to be financially conscious of their utilization decisions.[41]

Accompanying these gains for payers, aggregate-level savings to the overall system would come through the discipline of the free market. Since the amount left over in the account can be kept by the patient, he or she has a direct financial incentive to engage in the judicious use of medicine. In so doing, aggregate medical costs will be driven downward due to the price discipline of real free-market reforms.

Market Reform Purists argue that the use of such accounts would also address several related problems. First, it would erase the incentives created by deductibles (even relatively small deductibles) for low-income workers to forgo early intervention procedures but to spend unwisely once the deductible has been met. These incentives would be eliminated, since the MSA would cover initial costs and there would be a direct incentive to spend it judiciously throughout the year.[42] Second, the portability problem currently created when employees switch employers or lose jobs would be rectified, since any accrued funds would be kept by the individual employee to cover future health care expenses.[43]

The concept of Medical Savings Accounts had its origins in and finds support from the ranks of free-market ideologues. However, some members of organized medicine are also starting to advocate MSAs as the best means of preserving fee-for-service medicine. For instance, former AMA president Lonnie Bristow stated in a recent letter in the *New York Times* that in order to improve quality and access to care, "the only competitive option being considered by Congress that can satisfy your call for market-driven efficiency is the Medical Savings Account."[44]

With the prospect of large cost savings, the idea of Medical Savings Accounts has generated increased interest among policymakers. As of 1996, members of Congress were considering several proposals to adopt MSAs as a measure in health reform. In addition, a number of states have begun experimenting with them, and several private firms already have adopted them, though the tax changes which require federal legislation have not been implemented.[45]

EXPLICIT RATIONERS

"Explicit Rationers" make up the third group highly critical of the morality of managed care arrangements. These advocates share the familiar concerns about the ethical dilemmas which are created for physicians when they are placed under pressures to implicitly ration health care, whether for the sake of other patients or for the goal of returning profit to shareholders.[46]

As the name I have assigned them denotes, Explicit Rationers do not advocate a return to fee-for-service medicine. In addition to expressing concerns about over-utilization, Explicit Rationers assert that fee-for-service medicine is suspect from a moral standpoint because of its exclusive concern with the well-being of individual patients in an age of fiscal scarcity. Such an exclusive focus results in an unjust distribution of health care because some members of society use up as much of this scarce commodity as possible without considering what is left over for others. These commentators argue that given limited resources, the principle of exclusively focusing on individual patient needs has outlived its privileged place in medicine, and the health of the broader community must also receive significant moral consideration.[47]

Unlike other critics of managed care, Explicit Rationers propose options allowing for the influence of considerations that are external to the ideal patient-physician relationship in health care decisions. However, these influences are much different than those employed by managed care organizations.[48] These observers would like to see our health care system more closely resemble that of other nations where health care is directly rationed.

Explicit Rationers suggest various methods by which specific priorities for allocating care could be established. First, commentators such as Daniel Callahan have suggested that rationing could be accomplished by age. This criterion relies on the idea that at some point, the old should die gracefully. After a specific chronological point, medicine should not be used to extend life.[49] Others who advocate this criterion have pointed to the age-related rationing example set by the British model. While the British approach is not technically an explicit rationing plan, a far greater proportion of limited health care resources is spent on children than adults.[50]

Second, rationing could be accomplished, at least in part, by "sin exclusions," which would limit care based upon lifestyle choices within the realm of individual volition that place health at risk. This proposal proceeds along the line of reasoning that those who willingly engage in behavior which jeopardizes their own health have no right to receive priority for scarce resources. For example, those who have played a major role in the demise of their own health through smoking, obesity, or drug or alcohol abuse would be placed into low priority positions for high-cost treatments.[51]

Third, priorities could be established through the process of community discussion in which categories of injury and disease are ranked so that funding for treatments may be allocated accordingly. This was the approach of the recent Oregon Medicaid plan.[52] Within such a proposal, quality-of-life distinctions are considered in the establishment of rankings, since various ailments need to be weighed against each other to determine the greater priority.[53] In addition, prioritization would be based upon strict assessments of the value of particular procedures through quality and outcomes research. Medical "cookbooks" which entail the development of strict practice protocols for treatment and the linking of reimbursement with outcome would be formulated.[54] In conjunction with quality-of-life assessments, patients would then be triaged according to the degree of cost versus effectiveness of the treatments they need.

To be sure, community rankings could also be used to establish fixed limits in a top-down approach to rationing. This is similar to the British system, in which a global budget is set and physicians are forced to operate within it. In effect, this system rations care by limiting resources such as the availability of hospital beds or MRI scanners to physicians, which forces doctors to make trade-offs and to be more selective in deciding who is to receive care. However, such a model is really an *implicit* rationing plan and, on the surface, bears many structural similarities to managed care arrangements, since physicians are placed in the position of making allocation decisions. Because of its nondemocratic nature, proponents of explicit rationing would reject such a model.

Regardless of how rationing criteria are established, those who support the use of *explicit* rationing standards argue that preestablished priorities would protect physicians from the ethical dilemmas created by current managed care arrangements, which force them to make implicit, ad hoc rationing decisions at the bedside. Since resources are limited, proponents of this method of reform contend that it is clear that rationing must take place. However, from a moral perspective, such decisions are not ones that physicians should be expected to make. They should not be placed in the ethically untenable position of attempting to serve as the patient's advocate while simultaneously holding the line on costs.[55]

In response to the moral concerns of those who disdain the mere mention of the term "rationing," supporters of explicit rationing plans argue that we as a society have always rationed health care in some manner, though it is hidden in the current system.[56] Since the demand for health care exceeds the supply, rationing has and always will take place. Under current models, medicine is actually rationed in favor of those who can pay for it because society allows cost to be used as a determinant in accessing care.[57]

Explicit Rationers argue that managed care arrangements are really *implicit* rationing schemes with global budgets set by third-party payers. Doctors make treatment decisions with these parameters in mind.[58] Thus, Explicit Rationers are morally concerned about the nondemocratic method by which managed care arrangements make rationing decisions, since so much is hidden from the patient.[59] They contend that making these decisions consciously and openly is a better approach from a moral standpoint, since it would invite those most affected by such decisions to join the discussion. We as a society should take responsibility and acknowledge that the time has come to consciously make these types of decisions. The community should explicitly make rationing choices rather than allow the market or managed care organizations to insidiously do society's dirty work.

Explicit rationing plans would clearly curtail patient and physician autonomy. However, preestablished priorities, rather than the incentives used by managed care organizations, would place limits on patient treatment decisions. While the development of preestablished priorities through the community, as in the Oregon model, can be viewed as an extension of the "self" (in a political sense) rather than a third party, it is clear that explicit rationing shifts the focus from individual well-being to that of the broader community. Although this may not be a "third-party" influence in a technical sense, the practical effect is similar: needs other than the health of individual patients are significant factors for consideration. Thus, Explicit Rationers can be placed in the lower-right quadrant of Diagram 1.

Three Reframing the Debate

Perspectives in Support of Managed Care

In contrast to the three "types" opposing of managed care, three "types" in the current debate support managed care as the most ethical course of health care reform: the For-Profit Managed Care Champions, the Non-Profit Organization Supporters, and the Cautious Supporters of Managed Care. While there are disagreements among them with respect to particular aspects of managed care, they also share a tremendous amount of common ground.

ARGUMENTS IN COMMON

Like Explicit Rationers, supporters of managed care argue that in an age of fiscal scarcity, strong measures must be taken to curb rising costs, thereby ensuring that health care remain affordable for members of the broader community.[1] However, they believe that explicit rationing schemes are politically and practically unfeasible because they negate the clinical freedom that the practice of medicine demands.[2] Consequently, they argue that it is only within managed care "that one can find the economic discipline produced by a fixed resource limit for caring for a defined population."[3] Managed care is characterized as the only system that offers a unique combination of low out-of-pocket costs, improvements in quality, and the coordination of care so that minor illnesses do not develop into more serious ones.[4]

As an alternative to explicit rationing, advocates of managed care embrace market-*oriented* reforms and incentives for cost consciousness. They argue that such measures represent the only means to rein in exploding costs, through cutting unnecessary procedures and tests, while maintaining the necessary flexibility for physicians to properly practice medicine.[5] With lower costs, accessibility will increase for the estimated 37 million Americans who currently have no health coverage at all.[6] Although the relationship between physician and patient will be less than ideal, supporters of managed care note that given broader access, more people can have such a relationship in the first place.[7]

Like Market Reform Purists, supporters of managed care point to the fiscal irresponsibility of fee-for-service arrangements covered by traditional indemnity plans, under which patients are so far removed from the actual financial outlays that they are said to be "cost-unconscious consumers." Proponents of managed care cite studies, including the previously mentioned Rand Corporation series, in order to sustain their argument that market competition will serve to quickly cut the fat out of the system. Several studies have concluded that 20 to 30 percent of all medical procedures are probably wasteful.[8] As a more specific example, advocates of managed care point out that many procedures, such as electronic fetal heart rate monitoring, have become standard before their value has ever been proven.[9] The widespread employment of these procedures has resulted in the consumption of resources that could have been used in other areas of need.

Instead of primarily focusing incentives on individual patients (as advocates of Medical Savings Accounts do), those who favor managed care reason that since physician decisions account for an estimated 75 to 80 percent of total health care expenditures, this is the best place to target cost-control incentives.[10] Proper incentives aimed at physician decisions, they assert, are the only means whereby costs can be contained while preserving the power of doctors to make the medical judgments.[11] These mechanisms are the only real alternative to "cookbook" approaches to medicine incorporated within explicit rationing schemes.[12] While patients are also given financial incentives in managed care, these incentives are aimed at encouraging the patient to use providers in the contracted network, rather than to negotiate prices directly with physicians.

On a related note, supporters of managed care argue that market competition utilizing managed care organizations is much better than the alternative models at efficiently deploying resources, by avoiding the duplication of expensive technologies and determining the number of physicians and specialists that are truly needed. For example, some estimates state that if the country functioned with the same doctor ratio as Kaiser, we would need only 320,000 doctors compared to the nearly 700,000 we have today.[13] They claim that some additional benefits of managed care will be higher quality by means of rigorous reviews of standards and a greater emphasis on lower-cost treatments.[14]

In response to criticisms that managed care endangers patients, its supporters answer that much of the moral concern over damage to individual patient well-being is overstated and relies on anecdotal rather than empirical evidence.[15] They argue that managed care mainly eliminates unnecessary procedures or procedures of questionable clinical value, and thus, cost-reductions reduce the quantity but not necessarily the quality of care. As evidence, they cite several recent studies showing that cost savings do not have a noticeable effect on quality.[16] Furthermore, they point to data reported by the American Medical Association that 85 percent of all HMO physicians are board-certified compared with 61 percent of physicians nationwide, as further proof that managed care is "a quality driven system."[17]

In addressing concerns that managed care creates financial conflicts of interest for physicians, proponents of managed care respond in several ways. First, they point out that there is no payment system that is free from conflicts of interest of one type or another. Freedom from such dilemmas under fee-for-service medicine, the model to which Patient-Centered Purists wish to return, is really more myth than reality.[18] Conflicts of interest are not unique to managed care plans, since there is already a clear temptation for physicians under fee-for-service arrangements to profit through the practice of over-prescribing.[19] Moreover, in some situations under fee-for-service arrangements, the costs of a procedure may outweigh the benefits, placing an unnecessary financial burden upon the patient, thereby raising health care costs for all, and contributing to the problem of fiscal scarcity.[20]

Managed care advocates also note that over-utilization can lead to more than just financial conflicts. Iatrogenic harm (harm resulting from unnecessary tests and procedures) may be an unintended consequence.[21] Michael McGarvey contends that the Hippocratic exhortation *primum non nocere* is far more likely to be violated by overtreatment than by undertreatment.[22] Even a salary-based remuneration system is subject to abuse. Salaried physicians may be tempted to underserve patients, through scheduling fewer follow-up visits, performing fewer procedures, or focusing on other activities, such as research, to generate additional income.[23]

Finally, managed care supporters assert that the mere presence of financial incentives to cut costs does not necessitate a conflict of interest. Some contend that professional norms and the possibilities of malpractice suits are sufficiently strong restraining forces against abuse.[24] E. Haavi Morreim argues that physicians can act as agents of the patient and of cost control as long as they disclose the financial constraints under which they operate.[25]

FOR-PROFIT MANAGED CARE CHAMPIONS

The first, and most often cited, perspective in support of managed care is held by those whom I have termed "For-Profit Managed Care Champions." In general, supporters of this position believe in the strong use of the free market, especially the profit motive and financial incentives, in managed care arrangements in order to encourage efficiency in health care decisions. As such, they can be placed in the upper-right quadrant of the typology (Diagram 1) developed in the previous chapter.

Advocates of profit-seeking managed care organizations utilize many of the arguments for distributive justice and cost-containment advanced by other supporters of managed care. They too argue that market-based competition through managed care is the most efficient means of reducing soaring health care costs by providing incentives to reduce wasteful procedures.[26] However, these advocates, such as Malik Hasan, chairman of Health Systems International, the parent company of Health Net, favor more extensive uses of the market mechanism than do other supporters of managed care. Hasan has stated that specifically *for-profit* organizations are best suited to the new health care environment.[27] He has argued that the profit motive has helped managed care companies attract the best executives, who in turn have applied corporate strategy techniques to compel greater efficiency in the system.[28]

"For-profit" advocates point to data showing that only since the growth of for-profit organizations has the rate of increase of health premiums dropped below inflation, for the first time in a decade.[29] Such savings, these supporters contend, which have come through factors such as the consolidation of facilities and lowering of fees charged by specialists, are gains that could not have come without the unleashing of the power of the free market to correct inefficiencies.[30]

Supporters of for-profit organizations, responding to accusations that the profit motive and return to shareholders will damage patient care through immoral incentive systems to doctors and unconscionable utilization review decisions, reply that these concerns are unwarranted. They argue that the assumption that businesses seek only short-term profits is a false one.[31] Expressing faith that current regulations and the marketplace will punish unscrupulous actors, they claim that health care organizations must satisfy their customers in order to achieve long-term success. Moreover, they argue, it would make no sense from a financial standpoint to skimp on quality, since a sicker patient will cost more to the plan in the long run.[32] Physicians can also insure themselves against the financial costs of sicker patients, thus further discouraging the withholding of care.[33]

One industry lobbyist echoes these claims by pointing out that in California, fewer than 2,000 complaints are filed against HMOs each year, a good record considering that there are 12 million members in that state alone.[34] While many people are enrolled in non-profits, the majority of patients are now members of plans offered by for-profit organizations. Thus, there are relatively few complaints against for-profit MCOs. Supporters also argue that the industry is already policing itself. The National Committee for Quality Assurance, a private body governed by employers, managed care industry officials, organized labor, and a consumer representative, is developing voluntary standards for quality determination and accreditation for HMOs. The association is relatively new (and there is some suspicion that it is an industry mouthpiece), but the fact that some employers are already requiring accreditation from this organization for the health plans they use is offered as evidence that the market has built-in restraints.[35]

For-Profit Managed Care Champions further argue that for-profit plans are not profiting as a result of reductions in the quality of care, but because they are meeting a burgeoning demand for lower health care costs.[36] They assert that the current emphasis on efficiency is not purely profit-driven but rather a response to public concern and economic demand for lower costs in medical care. Thus, many of these cost-cutting practices would exist regardless of the profit motive.[37] However, since these organizations have been successful at providing lower cost premiums to purchasers, they deserve a fair price for their efforts.[38] Uwe Reinhardt has offered a defense of profit-making by managed care organizations on the grounds that they have successfully reversed the trend in health care costs, something no other entity has been able to accomplish.[39]

In response to criticisms of the current level of profits, For-Profit Managed Care Champions predict that high margins will decrease over time as competition increases, saving money for patients and trimming the fat out of the system. In addition, they claim that in the long-run, price competition will drive out the weakest firms. Over time, this will force competition on the basis of benefits and quality of care, giving patients and their physicians strong bargaining power and restoring them as the primary decision makers.[40] They note that because premium costs are not keeping up with inflation, corporate profits are already on the decline.[41] In fact, a growing number of employers are demanding quality and accreditation reviews precisely because industry consolidation makes many plans almost indistinguishable in terms of price alone.[42]

These arguments justify profit on the basis of efficiency. Some advocates of for-profit organizations also employ liberty-based perspectives to defend the corporate ownership of health care institutions and the profit motive in health care. This line of reasoning can be found in H. Tristam Engelhardt Jr. and Michael Rie (commenting on medicine as a whole "industry," not specifically on MCOs), who argue that although it is "morally praiseworthy to care for the ill without thought of recompense," for-profit medicine is ethical because it "comes into being through the free choice of consenting adults."[43]

Relying on such "contract" reasoning, Mark Waymack argues that cost-containment measures and the denial of expensive benefits are problematic, but they do not necessarily present an "*ethical conflict for the reason that the consumer has willingly chosen to participate in this kind of health plan.*" Waymack reasons that this is the cost of choosing to purchase coverage that is equivalent to a "basic model of a Ford automobile" rather than "the elegantly appointed Mercedes." If a consumer chooses the lower-cost automobile model, Waymack argues, that "he or she cannot accuse Ford Motor Company of acting unethically, even if the personal injury results as a consequence of the accident."[44] Similarly, if patients choose less expensive health care insurance, they should not expect remedies for which they did not pay beforehand. He also states that treating medicine as a business actually contributes to patient autonomy, with regard to allowing freedom of choice in "how much of one's resources to devote to health care insurance."[45]

Supporters of for-profit managed care organizations also argue that despite a few well-publicized miscues, most enrollees in both non-profit and for-profit managed care plans are highly satisfied with the services provided by their policies. For example, a *Los Angeles Times* survey reported very high satisfaction rates among all plan enrollees: 92 percent of those polled described their health care as good or excellent.[46]

In addressing concerns that capitation payment arrangements skim the economic cream by ushering in the demise of cost-shifting for indigent care, some advocates of for-profit managed care answer that this actually represents a positive consequence. In effect, they argue, this ends a practice that is immoral to begin with, since cost-shifting is a hidden form of taxation without representation.[47] In response to allegations of "cherry picking" or the complaint that HMOs attract younger or healthier patients, they state that research does not provide definitive data on this question.[48]

Finally, advocates of the profit motive in health care point out that seeking profit is not necessarily incompatible with an altruistic view of medicine as a public good. For example, Engelhardt and Rie point out that for-profit medicine is compatible with a single-payer system, and advocates of profit-seeking models do not necessarily reject a dedication to the selfless practice of medicine.[49]

In terms of legislative reform, For-Profit Managed Care Champions reject key elements of legislation along the lines of the Patient Protection Act discussed in chapter 1. In particular, they allege that such legislative measures represent a hidden means of protecting the financial interests of physicians, who are seeing the erosion of their previously unchecked professional dominance. They argue that restrictions that would limit the ability of managed care organizations to hire and fire doctors and offer care through closed panels will greatly increase premiums to patients.[50] Echoing these concerns, some employers defend the viability of managed care organizations by arguing that greater legislative restrictions will drive up their insurance benefit costs. For example, The Texas Business Group, an employer coalition, lauds the cost savings that HMOs have provided to employers in their criticisms of state-level versions of the Patient Protection Act.[51]

In general, supporters of for-profit managed care are opposed to large-scale legislative reform proposals, such as closing the ERISA loophole mentioned in chapter 1. They argue that this will encourage a rash of lawsuits and drive up employers' legal and health care costs "without improving care or even providing greater benefits."[52] They are extremely vocal about maintaining most of the cost-savings tools of their industry. However, probably for public relations reasons, they have not fought publicly or with much resolve over the imposition of minimum hospital stays for mothers of newborns and the removal of gag orders.

NON-PROFIT ORGANIZATION SUPPORTERS

The second position which supports the ideals and goals behind managed care is held by those whom I have termed "Non-Profit Organization Supporters." Adherents to this perspective support some degree of competition in health care in order to encourage efficiency, but reject a pure form of market discipline in which shareholder profits are at stake. They believe that the profit motive creates additional pressures on physicians by introducing share-holders into the equation, thereby further dividing physician loy-alties.[53] For example, Kate T. Christensen argues that in order to be ethical, managed care organizations must be chartered as not-for-profit.[54] As a result of these views, proponents of this viewpoint fall in the center of the lower-left quadrant of Diagram 1.

It is important to recognize this perspective because in the cur-rent debate, many people confuse the *concept* of managed care with the *organizational* form in which it is delivered. For example, in decrying the divided loyalties and greed created by the profit-seeking motive of managed care organizations, many observers seem to forget that a number of them are chartered as non-profit entities.[55] This mistake recurs both in popular forums and in the scholarly literature. Consequently, the perspective of supporters of the exclusive use of non-profit organizations serves as an impor-tant reminder that advocacy of some of the cost-saving mecha-nisms and procedures of managed care should not be confused with an endorsement of stockholder-owned corporations as the dominant model for delivery.

As the name I have assigned them indicates, Non-Profit Organi-zation Supporters accept the ideals and practices of managed care but reject the use of profit-seeking organizational models in its de-livery. For instance, in a recent editorial in the *Journal of the American Medical Association*, Carolyn Clancy and Howard Brody seem to take this position when they contrast "Jekyll care" with "Hyde care." They condemn plans in which "profits are returned to sharehold-ers" and praise those that utilize cost-effective procedures and in-vest earnings "in improvements in patient care."[56] Similarly, while acknowledging that managed care is not evil by nature, Arnold Relman argues that we as a society should be concerned about medical institutions that are run for the primary benefit of share-holders, on the grounds that medicine "cannot meet its responsi-bilities to society if it is dominated by business interests."[57] He reasons that the dilemma presented by for-profit health care is not just a conflict between the patient and social goals, but a conflict between the patient and the organizational goals of profit.[58]

Non-Profit Organization Supporters believe on moral grounds

that the cost savings achieved by managed care should not be distributed to shareholders. They agree that bedside rationing must take place in order to conserve resources, but it is morally acceptable only if the conserved assets are used to treat other patients or to conduct medical research that will benefit future patients, rather than to pay out profit on investment to shareholders.[59]

The "medical-loss ratios" of some for-profit organizations are frequently cited as evidence that sound ethics demand the exclusive use of non-profit organizations. These figures measure the percentage of revenues directly spent on patient care.[60] The low figures of some for-profit models are interpreted to indicate that too high a percentage of financial resources is being diverted for the purposes of salaries to executives, profit to shareholders, and administrative costs such as advertising used to attract new subscribers.[61]

Adherents to this perspective believe that non-profit chartered organizations facilitate the delivery of medicine in a manner that is more consistent with the traditional patient-centered norms of medicine.[62] Some also ground their moral arguments in a community-based philosophical approach to health care. They argue that medicine is fundamentally a public good rather than a private one. Thus, the fact that we allow corporations and their shareholders to profit on something that is such a fundamental human need speaks poorly of us as a moral community. For example, the late Cardinal Joseph Bernardin and others have expressed moral reservations about reducing medicine to the realm of other commodities such as hair spray and compact discs. While the profit sector has a viable place in society, Bernardin argues, medicine should not be a part of it.[63]

In terms of their perspectives on policy measures, Non-Profit Organization Supporters hold that managed care should be delivered mainly by two types of organization. Some prefer the older non-profit "staff" or "group" model organization, such as Kaiser, which had its origins in a sense of social mission, paid physicians on the basis of salary, and did not distribute profits to shareholders. They favor this model on the belief that this type of organization is under the least pressure to engage in the current practices that have raised social concern.[64]

Others, such as Relman, support non-profit community-based groups that would "minimize or avoid price competition" and would be physician-owned and operated.[65] These institutions would be technically non-profit since no shareholders would receive distributions. In theory, this would place trustworthy physicians who are guided by professional norms, rather than bureaucrats guided by the profit motive, in control of the practice of medicine.[66] The AMA and other organized medical associations are pushing for anti-trust relief in various legislatures so that physicians can start practices which would compete head-to-head with current managed care organizations.[67] Recently, a large coalition of employers in Minneapolis, which provides coverage for 400,000 employees, decided to bypass managed care organizations altogether and directly contract with a number of physician-owned groups for health services.[68]

CAUTIOUS SUPPORTERS OF MANAGED CARE

The final perspective defending managed care is held by those whom I have termed "Cautious Supporters of Managed Care." They support market-based reforms, yet simultaneously argue that strong regulations must be placed upon managed care organizations in order to protect patients from harm. Their fundamental claim is that the current problem lies not in the concept of managed care, but rather in how it is implemented.[69] Thus, they believe that while market-based reforms are the best course of action, the practices of MCOs should be limited in significant ways.

In contrast to "For-Profit Managed Care Champions," Cautious Supporters of Managed Care defend a more restrained market approach to health care. They can also be distinguished from "Non-Profit Organization Supporters" because they do not explicitly specify a preference about the tax status of the organizations involved in the delivery of care. However, they do contend that all managed care organizations must be bound by significant ethical responsibilities that go well beyond the mandate to maximize profit.[70]

Many physicians, albeit some by default, can be counted as adherents of this position.[71] Some physicians who actively opposed managed care have mitigated their positions, given the realities of its growth. These doctors seem to want to find ways to make the best of what they deem to be less than an ideal situation, by offering critical and cautious support of the newly emerging form of medicine.

In my view, this perspective is the most important one to identify in this debate. As noted earlier, much of the current literature, especially on the popular level, categorizes all supporters of managed care under a single rubric of market ideologues who wholeheartedly support all industry practices, including ones which may harm patients in the name of profit. When the perspective of cautious support is brought to light, we can see that arguments in support of market-based reforms should not be equated with an outright endorsement of *laissez-faire* medicine. Since I will develop this perspective in a more comprehensive fashion in the final chapters, I will offer only a brief description of it here.

In general, Cautious Supporters take the position that some of the criticisms advanced against managed care are overstated. However, they accept the validity of concerns about the potential for harm to patients and the broader society brought about by some of the more controversial practices. As such, they favor developing a more appropriate ethical model with which to guide the actions of these organizations. They believe that traditional medical and business approaches are both unequal to the task at hand.

In addition to urging the development of a moral paradigm, they also support more legislative and regulatory reforms to curb potential abuses by managed care organizations. For example, Alain Enthoven and Richard Kronick, the architects of the Clinton "managed competition" plan, advocate various safeguards to empower consumer choice and to address the "cherry picking" and portability problems associated with managed care.[72] Others assert that "gag orders" must be prohibited on moral grounds because these contractual provisions deny the amount of information available to consumers which is necessary to ensure some degree of fairness in transactions.[73]

In short, Cautious Supporters believe that market-based reforms are the only alternative to cost-inflating fee-for-service and impractical explicit rationing approaches to medicine. However, they sharply distinguish medicine from other commodities, since patients are at a significant informational disadvantage when purchasing health care. As a result, Cautious Supporters are concerned about harm caused by specific industry practices, and they support increased regulations of the industry as a solution. Cautious Supporters clearly advocate a much more limited free-market model than For-Profit Managed Care Champions. Thus, they fall in the middle of the upper-right quadrant of Diagram 1.

A simple dichotomy, for and against managed care, obscures the moral (and practical) issues of the managed care debate. The distinctions drawn by the six-part typology presented in this chapter and the last give us a clearer picture of the debate and enable us to appreciate the possibilities and the inevitable tradeoffs. The description of six distinct perspectives has laid the groundwork for a critical examination of the *validity* of each perspective, which is the task of the following chapters and is a prerequisite for seeking a moral framework for managed health care.

Four Fee-for-Service Medicine

The tragic situations presented by the popular media often foster the idea that managed care of any variety is a source of moral evil and that a return to non-managed care, identified with fee-for-service medicine, will cure these ills. This is the moral position of the Patient-Centered Purists, described earlier, who reject managed care in favor of a return to the dominance of fee-for-service arrangements and a reliance upon the professional ethical norms of medicine to safeguard the best interests of patients. They argue that the growth of managed care leads to the large-scale encroachment of market competition and business enterprises into medicine. This in turn destroys the ideal patient-physician relationship by turning health care into a mere commodity and furthermore, harms individual patients and society as a result of profit-seeking behavior.

As suggested earlier, many proponents of this perspective do not distinguish between for-profit and non-profit organizations in managed care. Presumably the distinction is unimportant because they reject the very ideals and principles behind managed care as a concept, regardless of the delivery model that is employed.[1] However, my suspicion is that some simply miss the distinction and unintentionally include non-profits among the targets of their attacks. Whatever the case may be, I include non-profit organizations in their rejection of "market competition" and the encroachment of "business" into health care.

In their descriptions of the threat that managed care arrangements bring to medicine, Patient-Centered Purists operate under the foundational belief that the worlds of business and medicine could not be further apart in terms of their moral objectives. Common statements to the effect that business and market competition will corrupt medicine, or that there are no business standards that would protect patients when financial demands conflict with medical goals, reflect this basic premise.[2]

While such sentiments are understandable, several operative assumptions are at work within them. Primarily, it is assumed that the "business ethic" is a corollary of the model proposed by Milton Friedman, which places the pursuit of profit within the limits of the law as the only goal of a publicly held corporation.[3] Unlike medicine, business is viewed as an arena with no ethical norms creating obligations beyond the fulfillment of explicitly made contracts. Employees of publicly held corporations are exclusively bound to maximize the wealth of their shareholders, giving little or no priority to the interests of consumers and other stakeholders.[4] Assuming this exclusive goal, the purists allege that patients will be hurt in a managed care setting since their interests will be necessarily subordinated to the pursuit of profit.

In contrast, Patient-Centered Purists assume that health care professionals are primarily motivated by altruistic concerns. Since they assume the "business ethic" is the corrupting influence on medicine, clearly they take it for granted that the prevailing "medical ethic" under fee-for-service is one in which the well-being of the patient is the sole consideration in making decisions.[5] The pictures of business and medicine created by these assumptions are completely antithetical. The image of business, and by association, of managed care, is one of "cowboy capitalism" in which the ethics of "purveyors" of various commodities rule the day. The image of fee-for-service medicine fits the ethos created by Norman Rockwell paintings of the charitable small-town doctor.[6] A natural consequence of these assumptions is the belief that the two paradigms should not mix, lest medicine lower itself to the corrupt sphere of business.

THE "BUSINESS ETHIC" ARGUMENT

Given the differences in how physicians and corporations are commonly portrayed, a dichotomistic view of these two arenas makes intuitive sense. However, such a conception fails to stand up to scrutiny. Several scholars have accurately noted that the assumptions made about the dichotomy inherent in the governing paradigms of business and medicine are greatly exaggerated.[7] Indeed, a deeper examination reveals that the realms of medicine and business are closer together than a cursory look indicates.

The description of the alleged "business ethic" relies on a narrow "custodian of wealth model" which assumes that short-term profit maximization is the only goal of business. Although some business transactions undoubtedly run along these lines, there are a host of competing descriptive and normative paradigms about business ethics and practice which challenge the accuracy of this model.[8] These alternative approaches reject the idea that a greed-driven *laissez-faire* model is best or that corporate officers are exclusively bound by fiduciary duties to maximize profits for shareholders.[9] I will offer an in-depth examination of one such approach, the stakeholder model, as a framework for managed care in chapter 8, and refrain from an extended discussion at this point.[10]

However, let us proceed for now on the assumption that corporations do exclusively operate within a narrow profit-driven framework. Even on this assumption, statements to the effect that there would be no room to favor the interests of patients when there are financial conflicts are exaggerated. Market-based competition has built-in restraints to regulate the behavior of managed care organizations to *some* degree. While it is clear that the free market does have pronounced limits as the sole governor of economic-related behavior, it has more capacity to protect patient interests than Patient-Centered Purists are willing to concede.

Profit-driven practices which coincide with patient interests are reactionary by nature and are not motivated by "pure" moral concerns per se. However, a business model based on self-interest can encourage such practices since they are compatible with a longer-term view of business.[11] This is evident in managed care, where market forces are already regulating the actors to some degree. For example, numerous studies confirm that some managed care arrangements aggressively treat patients to prevent higher costs from materializing.[12] These studies indicate that patients in HMO-model managed care arrangements are more likely to receive preventative care measures than patients outside HMOs. For instance, several studies, including one published in the *American Journal of Public Health*, reported that HMO enrollees were diagnosed at earlier stages for four types of cancer, and women were more likely to obtain mammograms, pap smears, and other life-saving treatments.[13]

Consistent with the functioning of any competitive market, the large-scale profits that have been the focus of much public scrutiny are unlikely to last. As competition increases, savings will be passed to consumers. There is some evidence that this dynamic has already taken effect to some degree: a few years ago, profits decreased along with premium prices.[14] In 1995, health care premium increases were below the inflation rate for the first time in ten years.[15] While this is not a positive contribution if lower premium costs are achieved at the expense of the quality of care, some researchers believe that as competition grows and prices converge, plans will have to improve quality of care in order to differentiate themselves to consumers.[16]

To be sure, such an economic model of market discipline only functions properly if the interests of employers, who are the *purchasers* of most plans, and those of patients, who are the *users* of health care, are aligned. While most critics view the possibilities of such an alignment as remote, since it is presumed that the sole priority of employers is to save money, a growing number of employers do appear to have concerns for their employees and are actively pursuing quality improvements. For example, numerous employers are voluntarily requiring accreditation from the NCQA, a private organization, for plans they adopt.[17] With plans to incorporate the NCQA standards, other large public and private employers have joined forces with the Health Care Financing Administration to form an alliance to rate and improve the quality of care delivered by managed care organizations. In total, this group is currently responsible for the purchase of health care for 80 million Americans.[18]

Market discipline is also forcing managed care organizations to address some of the notable concerns that have been raised about policies that may hurt patients. For example, in response to the demand for broader patient choice of doctors, several organizations are now offering multi-option preferred provider plans, where out-of-network providers may be used at a higher out-of-pocket cost to the patient. Some plans are allowing specialist visits without "gatekeeper" approval. Furthermore, as was highlighted earlier, the bad publicity in the deMeurers case led Health Net to revamp its procedures for decision making regarding coverage of bone marrow transplants. Within these new procedures, a pool of money has been set aside for treatments, and denials are sent to an outside agency, which in turn sends it to three independent experts. If one of these reviewers rules in favor of the transplant, it is performed.[19]

The point in raising these examples is not to establish that the market is the perfect regulatory force for health care, but rather to point out there is *some* room to favor a patient's interests within market-based managed care arrangements. Since corporations must consider a host of surrounding social demands in order to earn a profit, a longer-term view of business mandates that these interests be considered.

THE "MEDICAL ETHIC" ARGUMENT

Along with the overly negative assessment of managed care under the "business ethic" argument, Patient-Centered Purists regularly overestimate the sanctity of the traditional fee-for-service arrangement and the "medical ethic" under which it has operated. In so doing, these advocates extend portrayals of the altruistic small-town doctor to the entire medical profession. They assume that unlike "business," fee-for-service medicine has traditionally been dominated by proactive, ethically motivated behavior that favors patient health without much attention to financial matters.

While this portrayal of medicine is quite common, it relies in part on the premise that physicians are morally superior people.[20] To be sure, the argument here is not that doctors are inferior. There are certainly many physicians, as there are business people, who engage in heroic actions and whose ethical moorings would never allow financial considerations to alter the established practices of their profession. However, the belief that, as a profession, physicians can be completely trusted as the exclusive guardians of the health of patients is one that should be held loosely. Evidence that the real governing ethic behind medicine is closer to the presumed "business ethic" than initially meets the eye can be readily found on two levels: *individual physicians* and *organized medicine*.

Individual Physicians and Altruism

The image of the patient-centered altruistic doctor whose only interest is curing the patient, without regard for financial reward, merely obscures the self-interested behavior that has existed long before cost-control or profit-seeking corporations entered the scene.

Medicine has always been about someone's financial gain. Uwe Reinhardt has remarked that it matters little if such gain is defined by the terms "honoraria," "income," or "profit," since these represent merely semantic differences.[21] To some degree, medicine has always been a commodity. Unlike priests, physicians certainly do not take a vow of poverty and are usually very well compensated for their work.[22] The same *Los Angeles Times* article in which Lonnie Bristow decries the greed in corporate involvement in medicine states that he received $278,000 during the previous year as chairman of the AMA, while "spending about half the year on AMA business."[23] A recent investigative series in the *Los Angeles Times*, which criticizes managed care plans operating in California, stands out quite succinctly because it overlooks this unattractive aspect of medicine. One featured article, which opens with the story of a doctor who at one time took home $400,000 a year in salary and whose $70,000 Mercedes Benz was for sale, laments the fate of doctors who were fleeing the state because their incomes were decreasing due to managed care.[24]

Also notorious are the practices of some physicians who allow financial considerations to dictate whom they will choose to treat. These doctors refuse to accept patients who are either uninsured or are covered by Medicare, the latter because of maximum rate limits which Medicare establishes for reimbursement. Other doctors demand prepayment for expensive procedures such as surgery and refuse treatment without it. Reinhardt points out that in effect, physicians who engage in these practices directly "skim the economic cream."[25] It is important to note that such refusal is consistent with the AMA principles of medical ethics and with current legal standards, which state that physicians are free to choose whom they will serve. In addition, medical ethics and law allow a physician to sever a relationship with a patient if the patient runs out of financial resources, provided sufficient notice is given, even if the patient has not found another provider of care.[26]

While managed care organizations have received most of the bad press about greed, for allegedly viewing patients as the means to profit and for their strong-arm tactics, one recent lawsuit reveals similar motivations by physicians. In this particular case, a group of Texas physicians lost many patients when the patients' employers switched over to a managed care network. When they tried to follow these patients by joining the physician panel and were told that there were already enough providers, they sued Aetna for violating their "property rights" by taking away their patients.[27] Although this may well be an isolated episode, it is curious language for professionals whose sole interests lie in altruistically serving the health needs of the public.

Furthermore, it is a well-documented fact that the sanctity of the ideal patient-physician relationship in fee-for-service arrangements has been overestimated. Under that model, financial conflicts of interest among medical professionals also existed.[28] However, doctors could more easily hide financially motivated behavior since their interests were often aligned with those of their patients. To be fair, some observers who favor a return to fee-for-service medicine acknowledge that there is an incentive to overtreat patients under the older model, though they state that this is less problematic than under the newer methods of reimbursement.[29]

When closely examined, patterns of physician behavior give serious evidence of the "adventurer" capitalism that is so disdained by the rhetoric of organized medicine. In addition to a history of abuses, such as fee splitting, self referrals, and kickbacks from hospitals, there are other examples of patterns of behavior in which the actions of physicians are intimately tied to their own financial interests.[30] Several studies have shown that when physicians have a financial stake in a secondary facility, they give increased numbers of referrals to their patients for procedures done by such facilities.[31] As a result, patients and insurers are overburdened with unnecessary costs, and patients may suffer health effects from overexposure to procedures such as x-rays and other diagnostic tests. Similarly, several researchers have noted large variations in the use of various medical services by geographic region, without apparent differences in the demographics or health status of the populations, offering further proof that factors other than true medical need can influence decision making.[32]

Dan Brock and Allen Buchanan have pointed out that under the dominance of fee-for-service medicine, there were relatively high and rising physician salaries, high rates of growth in the number of doctors in the better-paying specializations, and the geographic maldistribution of physicians towards wealthier areas.[33] With respect to the latter, Reinhardt has remarked:

> Careful empirical analysis has established what was known to any cab driver all along: physicians, like everyone else, like to locate in pleasant areas where the money is to be had. Thus, our favorite areas have been said to be vastly overdoctored, while other areas, notably inner cities have been sorely underserved.[34]

These factors further confirm that we should be skeptical of what several observers call the "Albert Schweitzer or Mother Theresa" image of the ordinary physician.[35]

Through these examples, we can see that financial considerations have been a priority in medicine long before the emergence of managed care. Indeed, one could make a plausible argument that whenever money changes hands, the prospect of a conflict of interest is insidiously present. For example, even the seemingly innocuous statement, "make another appointment to see me next week," could present a conflict of motives if the physician is reimbursed for each service provided.

Organized Medicine and the Patient-Centered Ethic

Analogous to the self-interested actions of individual physicians, the behavioral patterns of organized medicine offer little evidence to support an idealistic depiction of the profession. Reinhardt has asserted that the tenet revered by the medical profession, namely, that piece-rate compensation (fee-for-service) is the *sine qua non* of high-quality medical care, is dubious. He states that in effect, the profession is openly declaring that "its members are unlikely to do their best unless they are rewarded in cold cash for every little administration rendered."[36] Similarly, the traditional stance of the AMA and other professional medical societies against reforms, including changes in Medicare and Medicaid which would have provided broader access to care, leads one to question the altruistic image of organized medicine.[37]

Several observers have remarked that the medical profession resists or accepts government and corporate involvement in health care, depending upon whether it perceives such involvement to enhance or diminish professional autonomy. With respect to government involvement, Giles Scofield observes that "the medical profession has decried 'socialized' medicine, but not 'socialized' research (The National Institutes of Health), or 'socialized' hospital construction (the Hill-Burton Program)."[38] Similarly, he notes that physicians have taken ambiguous stands toward the corporate practice of medicine. On one hand, they have not fought against legislation allowing them to form professional corporations in order to capitalize on favorable corporate tax rates. On the other, they have resisted oversight of their billings by third-party organizations, reasoning that this constitutes the "corporate practice of medicine."[39] Commenting on these types of behavior, Paul Fieldstein has claimed that the political activities of organized medicine are best explained by a simple economic model of self-interest.[40]

Several recent situations seem to offer concrete evidence of these allegations. According to some skeptics, legislative measures such as the Patient Protection Act described in chapter 1 are really "physician protection" acts in disguise and are actually against patient interests, since they serve the economic well-being of physicians foremost.[41] John K. Inglehart states that the Patient Protection Act "was largely engineered by state medical societies seeking relief for financially beleaguered physicians."[42] Furthermore, the flip-flopping of positions by the AMA with respect to a recent Medicare reform proposal that would usher patients into managed care arrangements seems to offer further proof of these assertions. The AMA was originally against the plan, but when lawmakers offered over $20 billion in relief in the form of guarantees that their reimbursements would not be cut as severely as first proposed, the association reversed course and endorsed the proposal.[43]

Included in the deal made with members of Congress were provisions that cleared the way for the establishment of physician-owned health maintenance organizations that could compete directly with insurance companies for a share of the patients.[44] Both the ardent negotiation for such an opportunity and the subsequent enthusiasm with which physicians are viewing their entry into the *business* of managed care as both owners and providers should provoke suspicions. It seems natural to wonder whether many of their earlier expressed moral concerns were indeed sincere, or if these concerns have now simply taken a back seat to opportunities for greater profit.

Despite the evidence that professional medicine has acted in a manner consistent with the economic self-interest of a professional guild, much of the rhetoric coming from both practitioners and scholars regularly overlooks it. There are still constant demands for a return to the mythical "medical ethic," while the "business ethic" is condemned as incompatible and corrupt. A letter from a physician published in the *New England Journal of Medicine* captures the spirit of this position quite succinctly:

> What has set medicine apart from other occupations is the moral authority that stems from its dedication to patient care. The physician has been the patient's advocate and defender. By agreeing to serve the interests of the insurance company, the HMO, or anybody other than the patient, we are giving up the moral high ground—the singleness of motivation that has generated the trust of our patients and society. When we cooperate with the managed care agenda, we are reducing ourselves to the level of business people—just doing our job, making a living, doing what we are told.[45]

In light of the evidence just presented, these remarks are dubious. It is rather clear that medicine has not been characterized by proactive, selfless behavior that serves the exclusive interests of patients.

Patient-Centered Purists tend to exaggerate the differences between fee-for-service and managed care and between the "business" and "medical" ethics upon which they are presumed to be respectively based. Similarly, Patient-Centered Purists exaggerate the negative effects of managed care organizations on health care quality.

First, the claim that financial incentives not only reduce the quantity of care, but also undermine patient health in the process, is a legitimate but unproven concern. Individual cases have occurred in which patients have been harmed, but the available evidence measuring the quality of care on a broader scale leans toward the conclusion that the care given is not inferior. Furthermore, with respect to this criticism, Patient-Centered Purists seem to contradict themselves. In judging that managed care is inferior care, they imply that quality of care can be identified. However, they simultaneously reject evidence that managed care is a quality-driven system on the grounds that information is not available to adequately measure quality or to accurately determine what it is that constitutes truly "needed care."[46]

In actuality, managed care organizations are currently seriously involved in the development of quality measures. Some health care economists point out that managed care is forcing the development of measurements for patient outcomes by conducting rigorous testing of the use of costly technology.[47] Several researchers believe that to a large degree, the survival of managed care organizations may depend upon measurable quality improvements in patient health, as cost becomes less of a factor in competition.[48] Indeed, some managed care organizations are pressing forward with research that studies quality and are undertaking ambitious initiatives to improve the health status of their subscribers. Such endeavors did not take place under the dominance of fee-for-service medicine.[49]

Some plans are supporting endeavors that review and reward physicians, based in part on how they treat patients and not solely on cost savings. For example, United Healthcare monitors the use of mammography to ensure that a doctor is not cutting corners by avoiding procedures that might be medically important.[50] Furthermore, the growing alliances of employers that have formed and are relying upon NCQA standards will only further put pressure on these organizations to uphold quality in their quest for cost-efficiency.

In fairness, most experts concede that quality measures are in their infancy.[51] The empirical studies that have been conducted so far on whether or not managed care diminishes the quality of patient health have yielded mixed results. In addition, these studies have some critical limits. Thus, we should exercise caution in applying the conclusions of these studies. Many of them do not account for important variables. For example, most of these studies measure fee-for-service medicine against *one* model of managed care delivery, health maintenance organizations. Given the fact that a modified form of fee-for-service is used by some managed care models, such as preferred provider plans, the limits of the studies are obvious. Moreover, these studies do not differentiate between the non-profit and for-profit status of plans. Thus, the results of such studies should be understood within the context of these shortcomings.

Evidence from several studies has cast managed care in a somewhat negative light. One recent study led by John Ware compared the physical and mental health outcomes of chronically ill adults, including elderly and poor subgroups, on the basis of enrollment in HMOs versus traditional fee-for-service plans. The study found that while outcomes did not differ for the average chronically ill patient, elderly and poor patients seemed to fare worse in HMOs than under fee-for-service.[52]

A study by Dana Safran and two other researchers comparing quality of care in prepaid versus fee-for-service health care systems concluded that while HMOs were better in terms of preventative care and accessibility, they were lacking in accountability, continuity, and comprehensiveness.[53] A study conducted by the Virginia Board of Health Professions confirmed the conclusions drawn from the Safran study and further found that patient satisfaction levels were lower for sicker patients in HMOs than for patients with "average" health care needs.[54]

Another study of Medicare enrollees with joint and chest pain reported mixed data in the care received by HMO and fee-for-service plan enrollees. Patients enrolled in HMOs who had joint pain were more likely to visit a physician and receive a prescription for medicine than non-enrollees. For patients with both chest and joint pain, those in HMOs were less likely to see a specialist for care, have follow-up visits recommended, or have their progress monitored. HMO enrollees with joint pain also reported less symptomatic improvement than did non-enrollees.[55]

In contrast to the conclusions drawn by these studies, however, the majority of the evidence, while still in its elementary stages, favors the claim that cost savings do not necessarily translate into quality reductions for patients. As mentioned earlier, several studies seem to indicate that managed care may actually encourage higher quality care. A Rand Corporation study found that HMO members experienced up to 40 percent fewer hospitalization admissions and saved up to 28 percent on health care costs compared to those enrolled in fee-for-service plans. The study concluded that the cost savings through lower hospitalization rates were achieved "without lower levels of health status."[56]

In another study which is often cited, Barbara Starfield and several collaborators found "no consistent differences in quality of care overall for patients in different types of settings and no consistent relationships between cost-efficiency and quality of care."[57] Similarly, an Institute of Medicine Study concluded that the impact of utilization management on the quality of care is virtually nonexistent.[58]

A study based upon data gathered from the Medical Outcomes Study, an eight-year-long project evaluating the impact of different insurance arrangements on quality of care, also reached favorable conclusions about managed care. This particular study, conducted by Sheldon Greenfield and several other collaborators, focused on patients with high blood pressure or diabetes. The study found that HMO enrollees had outcomes similar to those of enrollees in traditional insurance plans. Moreover, the report also concluded that results of care provided by internists and family doctors (typical "gatekeepers" in managed care settings) were not significantly different from results of care given by specialists, even though patients under the care of specialists used more tests and procedures. The study found little evidence to substantiate accusations that HMOs withhold services for people with higher medical needs such as chronic disease, nor did it find that there are marked differences in care for the poor and elderly. However, the researchers did caution against making broad generalizations from their research, since their data was based upon only two medical conditions and three different organizations.[59]

Even Arnold Relman, a vocal critic of profit-seeking managed care organizations, admits that most of the literature so far confirms that the quality of medical care in prepaid capitated plans is comparable to that received in fee-for-service plans. In fact, he cites a study by Braveman and several collaborators that showed that patients in prepaid capitated plans had the lowest incidence of appendeal rupture. He explains this surprising conclusion by stating that HMOs pose few financial barriers to seek immediate medical attention and many of these organizations provide 24-hour access to a primary care physician or nurse.[60] However, he cautions against an overly optimistic conclusion by noting that managed care plans are diverse in terms of their organization, management, ownership, and variety of populations they serve.[61]

OTHER CONCERNS

In addition to skepticism about quality, Patient-Centered Purists have also expressed concerns that market competition will lead managed care organizations to engage in a host of other short-term profit-seeking behaviors that hurt patients and the broader society on a widespread level. Some of these issues, however, are clearly not unique to managed care. For example, if the judge in the case involving Joyce Ching and MetLife was correct in reducing the scope of the suit to simple malpractice, it was the physician, rather than the system, that was at fault. Mistaken diagnoses by physicians can occur independent of the type of reimbursement arrangements employed.

Many other aspects of health care that are less than ideal existed long before the arrival of managed care. Even under fee-for-service, there were clear restrictions on the availability of medical care and the autonomous practice of medicine. Carolyn Clancy and Howard Brody state that some degree of rationing has always occurred in medicine. They assert that "physicians have always spent more time and energy (if not money) on the sicker, needier patients and trusted the other patients to understand and sympathize."[62] As such, managed care does not overturn a traditional ethic, it calls attention to what has always been an implicit feature of it.[63]

Similarly, Nancy Jecker notes that limiting access to treatments is not unique to managed care. Preexisting conditions have always been cause for more expensive coverage or for complete denial of insurance coverage.[64] She also points out that complete freedom to choose one's physician has been limited in the past to some degree, because some types of providers, such as chiropractors and midwives, have been excluded from coverage by traditional indemnity plans.[65] Moreover, many traditional health plans have excluded some procedures, such as infertility treatments, as "experimental" in nature.

Concerns about the practice of "cherry picking" by managed care organizations also warrant attention. These accusations, however, seem to rely almost exclusively on anecdotal evidence, including well-circulated tales of how MCOs hold meetings on the second or third floor to sell plans to seniors, thereby self-selecting only the healthier enrollees who can make it up the stairs.[66] Despite the clear financial temptation to exclusively enroll only healthy members of the population, there is a lack of conclusive evidence that "cherry picking" actually occurs on a widespread level. A Congressional Budget Office study notes that self-selection occurs to some degree, while another study conducted in 1995 indicates that there is little difference in the health of enrollees in HMOs versus traditional fee-for-service plans.[67]

Both studies used dated information (the 1995 study was based on data from 1987), bringing into question their present reliability, since the period studied represents a time when managed care was not the dominant force that it is today. In fact, there are good reasons to believe that, by its very nature, the explosive growth in managed care plans will lead to the enrollment of higher risk populations. Furthermore, Medicare and other health reform programs will likely force managed care organizations to enroll older and less healthy populations by making pre-screening illegal.[68] Thus, it is likely that self-selection through "cherry picking" on a widespread level may become a largely insignificant issue in the near future.

With respect to these specific concerns, it is also important to recognize that managed care organizations are easy targets for criticism; they can become the scapegoats for many shortcomings in medical delivery. Their "greed" becomes the source of blame for the need to cut aggregate-level costs. Many members of society seem to have the notion that if managed care organizations were removed from the loop, health care resources would exist in almost limitless abundance. Yet available resources are limited, and cost-containment would still be necessary in the absence of MCOs.

Managed care organizations tend to be blamed for decisions made elsewhere in the health care system, and are almost universally blamed when care is withheld. Policymakers and voters run a considerable risk of enacting misguided legislation if they fail to determine where some of these decisions are really made. Sandra Johnson points out, for example, that managed care organization policies or reviewers can be falsely accused for a restriction on care, "when the real culprit is the rules and policies established by another entity, such as a hospital responding to a managed care environment."[69] Culpability can also be misplaced in situations in which a "three-tiered" model of remuneration is used. In these arrangements, a physician practice group receives the capitation payment from the managed care organization. In turn, individual physicians may be compensated through salary or fee-for-service.[70] Decisions to deny care in these situations are probably being made by reviewers at the level of the physician practice group, rather than the managed care organization.

Managed care organizations can also be falsely blamed in situations in which individual physicians are remunerated on a capitated basis. While the payment may be too low in some cases, there are clearly situations where the physician has made an unethical choice. Johnson observes that sometimes the charge that good care is prohibited by the plan can be made by a physician to mask other interests, such as financial gain or the avoidance of responsibility for a particular treatment decision.[71] In addition, several observers have pointed out that there is no possible health care system without some incentive to either overprescribe or underprescribe. Thus, in many cases, individual physicians must choose the moral path rather than falsely blame the payment arrangement or the MCO.

Along these lines, it is curious that the MCO is almost always blamed when a specialist is not included on the panel of network providers. The nearly universal assumption is that the plan has excluded the provider, when the actual reason may be that the specialist chooses not to work for reduced rates as specified by the contract. However, no data is available on reasons for exclusion.

Similarly, the statement that managed care "places" doctors in tenuous moral positions victimizes them as hapless participants. Even though physicians will lose patients if they choose not to sign contracts, surely they can avoid some of those that "force" them into these situations. Not all managed care contracts are alike. Physicians, as patient advocates, should not sign contracts likely to place them into dilemmas in which their ethics are challenged. Doctors and hospitals can also purchase insurance against having a higher-than-anticipated share of patients who suffer from costly illnesses in their capitation pools.[72] Consequently, society should not be so quick to blame the managed care organizations in situations in which care may be withheld.

The point in raising these examples is not to exonerate the morally suspect practices of managed care organizations or to deny that such practices exist. Rather, it is to call attention to the fact that we should be clear on where to appropriately place blame before making blanket accusations against managed care organizations. The fault may lie in the practice of doctors or other entities who have interests besides patient well-being at heart.

CONCLUSION

The ability of fee-for-service medicine to meet the patient-centered ideal has been greatly exaggerated. Based upon the prevailing assumptions about patient-physician relationships under this older model, one would assume that most patients lose the ideal relationship with their physician once they enroll in managed care. However, the fact is that many people have never enjoyed the ideal patient-physician relationship that is so often used as the benchmark for health care reform proposals. John La Puma states that with managed care, "the biggest change in the patient-physician relationship is that more patients are likely to have one, even if this relationship under managed care is different and not ideal."[73]

Some proponents of a return to fee-for-service also fail to acknowledge the fact that this model has played a major role in driving up our aggregate health care costs. As discussed earlier, under fee-for-service arrangements, both patients and physicians are given every incentive to demand "everything available" on their own or a loved one's behalf, without consideration of what might be left available to other members of the community. Thus, this model simply exacerbates rising aggregate costs and accessibility problems. Furthermore, the whole prescriptive case for a return to fee-for-service medicine relies on a false assumption that there are *unlimited* medical resources available.[74] In general, Patient-Centered Purists argue that a moral approach to medicine must separate decisions about health care from the cost of delivering that care, a task which is clearly impossible in our current climate of pronounced limits on resources.

Based upon these shortcomings, the case against managed care presented by those who advocate a return to the dominance of fee-for-service medicine is implausible. One need not go as far as accepting Paul Fieldstein's premise that economic self-interest is the guiding principle of organized medicine, to reject the arguments of the Patient-Centered Purists. When evidence beyond the anecdotal is examined, it seems clear that many of the criticisms offered by Patient-Centered Purists exaggerate the case against managed care.

A cursory view of the criticisms of managed care offered by Patient-Centered Purists gives the impression that a return to fee-for-service medicine would free us from many of the ethical dilemmas presented in health care delivery. Indeed, much of the rhetoric found in the news media and in the popular debate reflects this assumption. Although it is understandable why patients do not willingly accept what appear to be compromises on the amount of health care that either they or a loved one receives, a return to the dominance of fee-for-service arrangements, given their shortcomings, is not a practical option for health care reform. Clearly, the fee-for-service model was never free from many of the concerns that are now being raised about managed care. In addition, fee-for-service arrangements do not meet the norms of distributive justice described in the introductory chapter. Market-based reforms seem to be a necessary means of achieving a more ethical, though still imperfect, system of health care delivery.

A case on behalf of market-based reforms for health care and for some degree of limit setting through managed care is still open to criticism from two fronts. First, Market Reform Purists, who assert that managed care abridges the discipline of free-market reforms since the end consumers are not the purchasers of care, can argue that we should use a *truly* free market approach rather than just a market-*based* one. Second, Explicit Rationers can claim that if rationing must be carried out, we should rely both on more democratic means and on much more explicitly stated criteria to accomplish the task.

AN ETHICAL CRITIQUE OF THE ARGUMENTS OF MARKET REFORM PURISTS

Market Reform Purists are critical of both the older fee-for-service model under indemnity insurance plans *and* the emerging managed care system. They decry the waste caused by incentives that have created an ethos of "cost-unconsciousness" under traditional fee-for-service plans. They also disapprove of the concept of managed care on the grounds that it does not go far enough in the use of free-market reforms. Market Reform Purists criticize managed care programs for directing cost-cutting incentives toward physicians rather than toward patients. They argue that supporters of managed care make the false assumption that patients are and will remain largely ignorant about the services they are receiving. As a result, the discipline of the free market that forces suppliers to respond to consumer wants is abridged because patients are not allowed to play an active role in health care purchase decisions. Thus, as one observer notes, we have a "sham marketplace" under managed care rather than a truly free one.[1] John Goodman sums up this perspective by stating:

> A model based upon patient ignorance, however, is unlikely to survive. Increasingly, patients will use the Internet and commercial computer services to tap into medical libraries and databases, discuss ailments with other network users, and follow diagnosis model decision trees. Thus, the best model for the future is one that assumes that patients will know as much as their doctors—not about how to practice medicine, but about what medical practice has to offer.[2]

Relying on this reasoning, Market Reform Purists argue that patients, rather than physicians, should be given financial incentives to regulate the use of their own health care. They believe that the best practical way to give patients the freedom of choice necessary to be true end consumers, as they are in other markets, is the use of Medical Savings Accounts (MSAs).[3] Market Reform Purists contend that this will provide a comprehensive solution to the problem of rising costs in the health care system. Patients will have direct financial incentives to be cost-conscious in their utilization of services since it will be, in effect, their own money, rather than their employer's or insurer's, that will be spent. Moreover, since physicians will now have to market their services directly to patients, competition on the basis both of quality and price will increase. The market mechanism will function in the manner in which it is intended, driving down medical costs and saving large sums on the aggregate level in the process. Further benefits of the use of these accounts is that patients will be able to freely choose their physicians, and the "portability" problem, caused by changes in employment, will be effectively solved.

The goals behind the use of Medical Savings Accounts are morally praiseworthy. Driving down aggregate-level costs, increasing patient choices, and solving the portability problem should be endeavors undertaken by any health care reform proposal. Furthermore, increasing patient awareness and responsibility should be encouraged in the current climate. Under contemporary standards of informed consent in clinical decisions, patients have a significant role in decisions of great clinical complexity. It would be consistent to give patients greater levels of involvement in expenditure decisions as well. While these are important goals, however, the use of MSAs alone is not a comprehensive solution to the current health care crisis. Proposals advanced by Market Reform Purists are faulty on several important grounds.

First, proponents of current models of MSAs place too much faith in the market mechanism. As stated earlier, the free market has *some* promise for health care reform, but it is more limited than Market Reform Purists presume. It is doubtful that the level of knowledge required to adequately regulate individual physicians can be acquired by patients, even with the use of medical libraries and databases. While it is true that patients have the means to become more knowledgeable with such tools, the question remains whether patients can function as equal parties to transactions with medical providers, as they are presumed to do in other markets. It seems clear that they cannot; medicine is in a category of goods and services that is markedly different from most other commodities. The special nature of medicine makes it difficult if not impossible for consumers, acting on an individual basis, to comparison shop or to discipline high-priced or low-quality suppliers by taking their business elsewhere.

In their role as consumers, patients do not come under the care of physicians in the same conditions as they do when they purchase other goods. There is a clear difference in knowledge and power between the physician and the patient. The gap will remain even with the use of new computer technology. Medicine is too complex to have all of its nuances captured by databases. Many cases are unique and require judgment calls by physicians. In many situations, patients are not even aware of what is wrong with them, much less of the therapeutic options for treatment. Thus, patients cannot be expected to acquire the "perfect information" necessary to properly regulate their interactions with individual physicians.

Furthermore, many patients need health care when they are ill and cannot be expected to have the time or energy to comparison shop for the best available deal. As a consequence, it would be extremely difficult for most patients to negotiate over the cost of individual procedures on equal grounds with their doctors. While inequities in knowledge in the market for other services may be present, the gap and the resulting consequences are usually much greater in medicine. To be sure, similar difficulties arise in regulating managed care arrangements. However, it is easier for third parties to regulate managed care organizations than to regulate almost 700,000 individual physicians.

Second, the employment of MSAs may erode trust in patient-physician relationships even more drastically than under managed care. Doctors will be placed in the direct role of salespersons who profit, in part, according to their ability to negotiate in situations in which patients comparison shop. One could imagine that the quality of care would be affected negatively; patients will have a difficult time placing trust in someone with whom they just directly discussed the price of something as sacred as their health. Conversely, physicians might have negative feelings toward a particular patient as they spend more and more time on a treatment for which they may have pre-negotiated a price, resentful that the patient "got the better end" of the bargain. While negative feelings can also occur in managed care arrangements, the blame is usually placed on the organization which does most of the negotiating for prices and fees, providing a buffer between the individual patient and his or her physician. Moreover, care is prepaid in many managed care models, eliminating bartering over price between patient and physician.

Third, adopting Medical Savings Accounts could preserve many of the inequitable elements of access to care under fee-for-service medicine and would thereby violate a key Rawlsian principle of justice. Kenneth Thorpe notes that the adoption of MSAs will very likely lead to

> the enrollment of low risks while leaving high risks in low-deductible fee-for-service or managed care plans. This provides a financial boon to low risk employees (in particular for the estimated ten to fifteen percent of the employed workforce that does not incur medical expense in a typical year) and a bust for high risk employees who face higher health premiums.[4]

Specifically, only those families that spend less than the amount placed into the account by an employer would have any financial advantages in the use of MSAs. Thus, it is likely that the sickest members of society will be harmed. Those suffering from costly illnesses will be left in low-deductible insurance pools. Consequently, these members of society are likely to see their costs skyrocket. The healthier members of the population who have the incentive to use MSAs will be "cherry picked" or self-selected out of the pool.

In receiving a tax-free bonus representing unused care, individuals with good health will be, in effect, removing from the system what used to go toward caring for those who were less healthy. While one could argue that some managed care organizations are guilty of the same practice, since profits are taken out of the system, managed care has done so in the context of slowing the rate of increase in costs and achieving efficiency gains for the aggregate system. The cost-savings abilities of MSAs, which have not been tested, are much more questionable.

There are, in fact, some good reasons to believe that MSAs alone could not achieve the cost savings promised by its advocates. Physicians are accorded high levels of respect, usually well-deserved. Patients need to maintain a good relationship with their doctors, and need to be treated immediately when ill. It is questionable whether many patients will be hard-line negotiators for the price of their own medical care. Consequently, price competition may not occur to the degree imagined. In the absence of a high degree of such competition, there will be few incentives to force the integration of health care delivery systems, which reduces the excess capacity and overabundance of specialists that have plagued fee-for-service medicine.

In addition, individuals purchasing health care services will be confronting a system in which current prices reflect discounts that managed care plans have negotiated with providers. It is quite unlikely that individuals will have the economic leverage to obtain similar savings. In order for individuals using Medical Savings Accounts to receive such discounts, they probably would have to work within an acceptable list of doctors and hospitals, the way managed care enrollees do now.[5] In order to achieve some degree of cost savings, one of the most important advantages of Medical Savings Accounts, namely, unlimited freedom to choose providers, would be severely restricted in the process.

Recent surveys of well-insured American families indicate that roughly 6 percent of households account for 70 percent of all health care spending. At the other end of the spectrum, only 9 percent of the expenditures were traced to 72 percent of the households.[6] Since only families who spend low amounts annually on health care will benefit by using MSAs, this plan would only target expenditures that amount to a small percentage of total health care allocations. It would not help in curtailing the majority of expenditures. While total spending might decrease, it would not occur to the extent predicted by advocates of MSAs. In fact, Thorpe notes that although the type of plan does influence spending, "there is no published research suggesting that higher deductible plans are more effective in controlling growth in spending compared with health maintenance organizations, other forms of managed care, or low deductible fee-for-service plans."[7] With these cost factors in mind, and with the number of baby boomers reaching the age where more expenditures are used for health care, it is likely that only a small and decreasing percentage of the population will realize the projected benefits from the use of MSAs in the future.

Finally, given the penchant of the American Medical Association to engage in political behavior that is economically self-interested, we should be wary of MSAs simply because factions of the AMA are now leaning toward supporting them. Lonnie Bristow's statement, cited in chapter 2, in which he encourages the public not to dismiss MSAs, offers some evidence that this position is attractive to members of the AMA. This would be an interesting change in posture in an organization that has over and over again vilified the commodification of medicine. In fact, Medical Savings Accounts represent the ultimate commodification of medicine. If past patterns of behavior are accurate indicators, one can reasonably surmise that these members of the AMA believe that such accounts are financially advantageous for doctors. Indeed, it is much easier to negotiate fees with individual patients, who may be ill at the time of their "purchases," than with large organizations who have much more power to extract savings.

For these reasons, the position of Market Reform Purists is faulty. The argument that we should jettison managed care in favor of Medical Savings Accounts so that the free market will exercise its discipline will do little to fix our current crisis. In fact, the use of MSAs may not have a significant effect on cost and efficiency at all. Moreover, it will probably make the sicker members of our society worse off, which would morally outweigh any cost savings that could be achieved. Market Reform Purists do, however, remind us that patients have an important role to play in taking active responsibility for wasteful spending and escalating health care costs.

A good case can be made that MSAs should be used in conjunction with managed care plans. Some employers are already beginning to combine these accounts with managed care or preferred provider plans. The use of lower-cost providers is encouraged because deductibles can only be satisfied if a network physician is chosen.[8] Such a combination would encourage a degree of patient responsibility that is appropriate for the health care arena. It gives patients more incentives to be involved in health care decisions than they were under the older fee-for-service model, yet protects them from the responsibility of acting as lay doctors. The portability problem would also be addressed, and the least healthy members of society would not be left in expensive low-deductible plans. Furthermore, managed care organizations can provide a necessary buffer so that a high degree of trust between patients and physicians is maintained. When managed care plans and MSAs are used in conjunction, the former eliminates some of the non-egalitarian aspects of the latter.

AN ETHICAL CRITIQUE OF THE
ARGUMENTS OF EXPLICIT RATIONERS

A case on behalf of managed care relies in part on the argument that the time has come to ration care in the quest for distributive justice. As such, it is open to criticism by Explicit Rationers, who state that such decisions should be made with more open democratic participation. Like many other observers of the health care reform process, they too argue that rationing has always occurred to some degree. Under the dominance of fee-for-service medicine, the standards for rationing were price and the ability to pay. Thus, Explicit Rationers argue that an open rationing program does not violate an older ethic of medicine. Rather, instituting such a program is to be honest about what has already been practiced, while simultaneously making the criteria more just for those who would not receive appropriate amounts of care otherwise. In addition, Explicit Rationers denounce the manner in which rationing is conducted implicitly by physicians in managed care arrangements. As an alternative, they believe that society should establish predetermined criteria that relieve physicians of the burden of making such decisions alone. David Orentlicher provides a good summary of the practical and moral arguments that physicians should not make implicit "bedside" rationing decisions.[9]

First, accurate rationing requires a breadth of information that an individual physician cannot assimilate. In making such decisions, a doctor would need to know the potential and duration of the benefit of a treatment for a given patient, the costs and savings of the alternatives, and how the savings would then be spent. Second, there is tremendous inconsistency in practice, values, and experience among physicians. Where one doctor may elect to place resources, another may choose the opposite. Thus, the simple preferences of individual physicians rather than defensible moral principles may be guiding the decisions over who is to receive care, and how much care. Third, those who favor such policies argue that physicians do not have the training or expertise required to make value judgments of the moral magnitude that rationing requires. Finally, if physicians become responsible for rationing decisions, this will greatly decrease patient trust, since patients will have reason to be suspicious over whether or not their best interests are being favored.[10]

In lieu of physicians making such decisions at the bedside, those who favor explicit rationing argue that doctors should be asked to merely implement rationing decisions made by someone else. This avoids placing doctors in a morally tenuous position. In such an arrangement, physicians can function in the role of patient advocates, since treatment limits would be externally imposed.[11]

As outlined earlier, various proposals have been put forth which favor the use of explicit rationing. These programs would base rationing decisions upon several criteria, namely age, "sin exclusions," and community-chosen priorities. While these proposals vary in how they would establish criteria, they share some important common values. All of the plans justify a high degree of external influence on the patient-centered relationship, and all would limit the quantity of individual care in the interest of a more just distribution of medicine. However, rather than accepting the typical managed care arrangement as the external influence, they favor specific rationing criteria to decide who should receive care, and what kind of care, when there is competition for limited resources.

Explicit Rationers make important contributions by pointing out the fiscal limits in our current medical system and the subsequent need to be judicious in the use of care. Moreover, their belief in greater societal involvement in acknowledging fiscal scarcity and discussing priorities merits support. The problem lies in their approach to priorities. A close look at current explicit rationing proposals shows that they employ criteria which are morally unacceptable and practically infeasible.

The proposal to limit care based on age, offered by commentators such as Daniel Callahan, is much too inflexible when different patterns of aging are considered. Chronological age is clearly an inefficient indicator of health and other general "quality of life" distinctions. Many people of an advanced age enjoy healthy and robust life styles. Furthermore, even from the purely utilitarian viewpoint from which this proposal is advanced, many older seniors are still contributing members of society. Consequently, the assumption that these citizens will overtax the limited resources in the health care system is false. Some of those who enjoy good health may have used very little of the limited resources of health care even at elderly age. The criterion of age as the critical factor in distributing health care may, therefore, violate the very goal of equity being aimed at, since these members of society may never use their "fair share" of resources. Moreover, Arthur Caplan points out that the cut-off age would have to be as low as fifty, since "there aren't enough people who are eighty or ninety years old consuming health care resources to make a big dent in the budget."[12]

Certain "sin" based criteria may be appropriate grounds for increased cost sharing, but they are insufficient for purposes of direct exclusion. Clearly such proposals neglect the fact that many behavioral risk factors, such as obesity, may be independent of a person's free choice.[13] This criterion also represents a dangerous "slippery slope." Few if any among us are without "sin" in terms of behavior that may jeopardize our health. Sports activities, driving over the speed limit, eating cholesterol-rich foods, or residing in heavily polluted areas are all examples of behavior that could be used as criteria to withhold care from patients in the event that exclusions for other "sins" do not conserve enough resources. Furthermore, even if consistent and acceptable behaviorally-based criteria could be preestablished, doctors in emergency situations would be placed into the tenuous position of triaging patients based upon moral judgments made without knowledge of all the relevant facts.

A model based upon community-established criteria and utilizing "outcomes research" to formulate strict protocols and determine priorities is faulty for several reasons. Medicine is of such a complex nature that there are possibly millions of rationing decisions that must be made in order to consistently apply this type of model. From the sheer volume of medical decisions alone, it would be impossible for community members to establish standards to provide clear guidance for each situation. Even if all situations could all be ranked, medicine changes at such a rapid rate due to technology that these priorities for treatment would probably be obsolete before they were issued.[14]

In addition, the medical "cookbooks" necessary for such a plan limit the individuality of care that is critical to the practice of medicine. E. Haavi Morreim notes that these protocols can lead physicians to overlook "a myriad of important, medical, social, and moral details."[15] She states that flexibility is essential to medicine "not just for those patients who don't fit the cookbook, but to permit patients' own values to shape their medical care."[16] There are many medical treatments and tests that rely on a host of factors for their efficacy. It would be difficult, if not impossible, to provide physicians with preestablished guidelines that would account for each possible variation in the balance of these factors in order to determine the degree or duration of benefit involved.[17] Certainly, continuing work on the development of such protocols and the use of outcomes research should be encouraged in the name of efficiency. In fact, as discussed earlier, many managed care organizations are engaged in the development of these types of measures. However, care should be taken to acknowledge their limits and to avoid overestimating their effectiveness.

Another weakness of this model is that the average patient must place a high degree of trust in the moral judgment and technical expertise of "community members." In attempting to establish rationing criteria, community members are expected to act as "lay doctors" and weigh medical situations that may be technically far outside of their grasp. In addition, one of the weaknesses of the community-based models is that they may lack true democratic participation. The Oregon plan has been criticized because approximately 70 percent of the people who participated in the process were health care workers or had some connection to the health care system.[18] Thus, the process was less open and democratic than the idea of a community-based plan would suggest. David Hadorn further notes that the human psyche would probably have difficulty accepting rigid cost-effectiveness analysis; it is difficult to stand idly by when a person's life is threatened and effective rescue measures are available.[19]

Given these weaknesses, explicit rationing proposals do not amount to an ethical solution to the health care crisis. However, since there are limited resources, some type of rationing must continue to take place. In addition, patient advocacy has never been absolute. Doctors have always had to manage a load of patients with fixed time resources.[20] Thus, it would be pointless to take issue with the concept of rationing itself.

If outcomes research and "cookbooks" could be improved to the point that they reflect the practical realities of medicine, and if lay persons could use such data to make almost certain judgments about the efficacy of treatments, explicit rationing would be the most just proposal. A community-based strict protocol approach would be the fairest solution to the health care crisis. Assuming true democratic participation, such an approach would permit community members rather than government bureaucrats, health care plans, or physicians to make rationing decisions for them. However, outcomes research and strict protocols will probably never reach such a point given the special nature of medicine.

Consequently, implicit rationing through managed care arrangements presents a much better model than explicit rationing for several reasons. First, in some situations it is simply impossible for anyone but physicians to make these decisions in any way other than as ad hoc bedside decisions.[21] Often it takes time to make the diagnosis and to arrive at value judgments following the protocols and priorities of the rationing scheme, time that both physicians and patients may not have. Second, explicit rationing schemes, especially ones based upon "cookbooks," do not retain the flexibility needed for proper clinical practice; the physician is often in the best position to have information regarding the patient's condition, and it is simply impossible to develop guidelines for every situation. In addition to the need for clinical flexibility, the physician may also be the most knowledgeable about patient and family preferences for conservative or aggressive care and the value placed upon future outcomes.[22]

Implicit rationing is not, however, without its share of weaknesses. Having physicians play a significant role in making such decisions is less than ideal from a moral standpoint. However, as Orentlicher insightfully comments, the argument favoring reliance on physicians for making rationing judgments is not that they are good or appropriate decision makers, but that there is no better way to make such decisions.[23]

A more specific argument against implicit rationing within managed care arrangements can also be levied. The contention could be raised that either a community-based global limits approach or else the British system, in which broad financial allocations are set by the government, should be followed if implicit rationing must be employed. The argument here is that the "community" or the government has a greater interest in protecting patients than do profit-making corporations.

While there might be some truth to this claim, the failure

of recent federal health care reform proposals suggests that the American public is not very willing to accept such sweeping constraints on its health care choices. In addition to raising reasonable suspicions that a governmentally-run system would be inefficient, such constraints would violate Rawls's principle of the preservation of the greatest equal amount of liberty possible compatible with what others possess. Non-governmentally run programs may well achieve greater efficiency while simultaneously preserving greater amounts of liberty, by offering various kinds of options. David Mechanic further points out that community involvement in allocation decisions under the British model is greatly exaggerated. He notes that many administrative matters of technical complexity are decided out of the view of the public and can be influenced by powerful special-interest groups who have more technical knowledge than other affected parties.[24]

Explicit Rationers are troubled by the fact that in a privatized managed care system, versus a publicly run system, profits are flowing out of the health care system and into the corporate coffers. While I will address this possible shortcoming in detail in the next chapter, it is worth observing here that profit may be an unavoidable component of health care, given the fact that medicine has always contained an element of financial gain.

A GENERAL CASE FOR THE
MORALITY OF MANAGED CARE

As David Thomasma has noted, the goal of any health care reform proposal must be to improve the quality of care for the individual while simultaneously reducing economic burdens on the populace and on third-party payers such as the government and employers.[25] In light of the shortcomings of each alternative outlined, it seems clear that managed care offers the most promise of meeting these goals. Each of the proposals offered by the three types that reject managed care represent insufficient solutions to the health care crisis.

Fee-for-service medicine is arguably the best means to ensure individual patient well-being. However, it clearly fails in the quest for broader justice, since it does nothing to reverse rising aggregate health care costs. In fact, this older model has done almost everything possible to facilitate the opposite trend. Furthermore, those who favor fee-for-service arrangements and the absolute patient-centered ethic rest their arguments on several dubious premises. First, these advocates base their claims on the assumption that resources are unlimited, since they assert that medical treatment decisions should never be weighed against cost factors. If resources are indeed limited, their whole prescribed program is faulty. Second, based upon narrow interpretations of the ethics of "business" and "medicine," they exaggerate the differences between fee-for-service arrangements and managed care. They have taken a far too narrow and pessimistic view of business, and a far too positive one of the medical profession. This has, in turn, falsely colored their arguments against managed care organizations. However, Patient-Centered Purists do remind us that it is critical that as much of the patient-centered ethic should be preserved as possible within reform measures.

Market Reform Purists who favor the use of patient incentives to increase true market discipline remind us of the importance of encouraging patients to take an active role in health care allocation decisions. However, proponents of this perspective place too much trust in the power of the free market to lower costs and improve the quality of care. Since patients cannot and should not be expected to meet a standard of the "reasonable consumer" similar to the standard expected in the market for other goods, their ability to make value judgments about quality and cost, and thereby to discipline suppliers in the most efficient manner, is highly questionable. The prediction for cost savings from proposals such as Medical Savings Accounts is further suspect. Moreover, the potential for "cherry picking" and the resulting damage to the poorest members of society is accentuated by the use of these measures. Thus, the proposals offered by Market Reform Purists have little potential for balancing the goals of individual patient well-being and broader societal justice.

Explicit rationing proposals offer important reminders about the limited fiscal resources in our health care system. These proposals are laudable because they value the broader goal of justice in terms of access to health care for more members of society. Supporters of these proposals make an important contribution by pointing out the need for patients to assume some responsibility in acknowledging that resources are limited, and in pointing out that health care should be viewed as a common good. However, these proposals are also morally and practically suspect because the specific criteria that would be used to prioritize health care services are questionable. At least several of these proposals rely upon an unrealistic portrayal of the nature of the practice of medicine for their success. In addition, under current conditions, explicit rationing plans reduce liberty too severely, especially when there are other viable options available.

In light of the weaknesses of the proposed alternatives, managed care is the model that offers the most promise in terms of achieving a balance of the previously mentioned goals of health care reform. Although it is still an imperfect solution, managed care offers the best hope of retaining as much of the patient-centered ethic as possible while lowering aggregate costs and thereby increasing the potential for improved access to care. Numerous studies confirm this. One study by Lewin-VHI Inc. reports that managed care arrangements of Independent Practice Associations produce 14 to 23 percent savings over fee-for-service systems with at least 10 percent of those savings accruing to the whole medical system.[26] Managed care has also encouraged numerous quality and outcomes studies that were never attempted under fee-for-service medicine.

Instead of a total free-market approach, managed care uses market-*based* reforms that do not leave individual patients with the burden of possessing the perfect information necessary to negotiate in the market. In lieu of explicit rationing schemes and a total free-market approach, managed care employs implicit rationing, which is a more appropriate model for reform since it retains the flexibility necessary for physicians to engage in the effective practice of medicine. While the use of capitation arrangements has received a tremendous amount of bad press, it may actually offer more freedom to the physician, while curbing aggregate costs, than other cost-containment measures.[27]

Nonetheless, the incentives used by managed care are subject to abuse because of the very real threat of undertreatment and other practices utilized in the quest for profit, both on the level of individual doctors and of organizations. Though profit is not their only goal, publicly held corporations do have financial obligations to shareholders. Upholding these duties could clearly conflict with patient needs. Consequently, several observers have supported managed care, but with some critical limitations. For example, some have argued that in order to be ethical, managed care organizations should be non-profit in nature. Others have claimed that for-profits are morally a better fit for today's health care climate. A third perspective is that all managed care organizations, regardless of tax-status, should have more legal and ethical restraints placed upon their activities. In the next two chapters, I will assess these perspectives in support of managed care.

Six   The Ethical Importance of the Non-Profit Distinction

Even though a case can be made for the general moral viability of the concepts and ideals behind managed care, significant questions remain over the place of the profit motive in managed care organizations. In fact, the ethical issue surrounding the tax-status of the institutions offering plans to patients has become one of the primary focal points of the current discussion. It is quite common to see statements to the effect that managed care organizations should be chartered as not-for-profit if they are to retain their ethical moorings.[1]

As described in an earlier chapter, a number of commentators have expressed concern about the possible detrimental effects of the emerging dominance of for-profit models. These observers fear that the explosive growth of these institutions will bring some of the most deplorable aspects of market competition into an arena that should be governed by altruistic concerns for the well-being of patients. Some critics have even asserted that the profit status of the organization is the *most important* moral difference among managed care institutions.[2]

Non-Profit Organization Supporters contend that the delivery of managed care must be through organizations which do not distribute profits to shareholders.[3] In their view, the goal of cost containment is defensible if the motive is one of societal justice in terms of a more equitable distribution of scarce resources. These observers argue that medicine is a "public" good and therefore should not be allocated based upon the whims of the private market. Earning profits on something as sacred as health care speaks poorly of us as a moral community on both concrete and symbolic levels.[4] Furthermore, adherents of this perspective believe that non-profit organizations are better able to serve the moral aims of patient advocacy and societal well-being because they have some significant advantages over shareholder-owned organizations.

These advocates claim that these advantages begin with differences in organizational *accountability*. They argue that physicians employed by non-profit entities are at much greater liberty to practice medicine according to the traditional patient-centered ethic. Since non-profit organizations are not accountable to shareholders, physicians are free from the direct pressures that challenge their counterparts in publicly-owned corporations to return financial gains on investment.[5] In for-profit institutions, financial obligations to shareholders further complicate the already tenuous physician-patient relationship by introducing an unnecessary set of interests into the health care equation. As a result, physician loyalties are divided further from the ideal of an exclusive focus on the needs of individual patients.[6]

The operational *motives* of the two types of organizations are also radically different. Contrary to profit-seeking organizations, the goal of non-profit models is patient well-being rather than the health of the bottom line. Any "profits" or "surpluses" in revenues attained by non-profits are mere by-products of the efficient practice of medicine rather than the goal itself. Phillip Nudelman and Linda Andrews of Group Health Cooperative of Puget Sound (a non-profit HMO) sum up this perspective well by stating that the major differences between the two types of organizations lie in "purpose, values, attitude, and behavior: a for-profit plan provides a service so it can make a profit; a not-for-profit plan makes a profit so that it can provide a service."[7]

Advocates of the exclusive use of non-profits argue that as a result of these differences in accountability and motives, plans offered by non-profit organizations will be distinguishable from their for-profit counterparts in terms of specific *behavior* that favors patient health. In particular, non-profit plans will perform better than their for-profit counterparts in the morally important categories of quality of treatment and societal accessibility to care. In non-profit plans, any funds taken in as revenues that exceed direct expenses are plowed back into the health care cycle for medical-related needs. In contrast, shareholder distributions in for-profit models directly extract resources from that which is available for health care. Moreover, large amounts of revenues are utilized for administrative and marketing expenses to enroll new subscribers.[8] Differences in Medical Loss Ratios (MLRs) are often cited to show that for-profits spend a lower percentage of their revenues on health care for their enrollees than non-profits.[9] Non-Profit Organization Supporters argue that lower quality of care in for-profit models is a direct consequence of these disparities.

For-profit plans will also, allegedly, hurt the poor by exacerbating accessibility problems. By extracting profits out of the system, critical resources applied toward the costs of indigent care through the traditional practice of cost shifting will be eliminated.[10] In addition, the competition these organizations bring will only serve to evoke the tendency of all managed care organizations to engage in practices that squeeze providers and "skim the economic cream" out of the health care system. Non-profit plans will be compelled to act similarly as a direct consequence, lest they be forced to bear the cost of indigent care alone.

These arguments offer what appear to be convincing and weighty moral reasons to oppose the participation of for-profit organizations in managed health care. After all, traditional beliefs hold that the practice of medicine should be motivated by altruism rather than by personal gain. However, upon further scrutiny, we can see that many of the claims about the disparities between these two models are overstated. In what is to follow, I will examine the foundational argument that non-profits must be used if we approach medicine as a community good, and compare the two types of managed care organizations in terms of their differences in accountability, motives, and specific behavior.

NON-PROFITS AND MEDICINE AS A COMMUNITY GOOD

The argument that health care plans should be offered by non-profit organizations, because gaining financially by providing medical care violates moral norms of distributing public goods, is intuitively attractive. There is indeed something morally appealing about approaching medicine as a form of social service, and the statement this makes about society as a moral community. However, such a perspective rests upon numerous assumptions that non-profits actually offer a superior conduit toward these goals.

One assumption is that the exclusive use of non-profit organizations will remove medicine from private marketplace transactions, which in turn will automatically lead to a more just distribution of health care. While it would be ideal if non-profits could give away care without thought of economic considerations, these organizations also operate with financial constraints within competitive environments. Market-oriented forces would still be present even if all managed care organizations were rendered non-profit in status. Thus, a more just distribution of health care will not be a necessary outflow of such a change. Non-profit organizations cannot afford either to operate without consideration of cost constraints or to give away significant amounts of free health care.

The notion that for-profits should be proscribed because profit and community goods are somehow mutually exclusive relies upon an assumption that the nature of private ownership of the means to distribution of a good necessarily prevents the community from having a significant stake in it. Such a conception is faulty because it relies upon a narrow Lockean understanding of human beings as atomistic individuals, which has ironically led to the "custodian of wealth" model of corporate social responsibility, in which business organizations are conceptualized as mere engines of economic efficiency. Clearly, private ownership and community morality are not so estranged.

For example, Dan Brock and Allen Buchanan draw a corollary argument about the distribution of food, another critical sustenance good. They note that there is no societal expectation that just because a profit is made on food items, grocery stores have a special obligation to give them away without recompense. However, the community has made provisions for the distribution of food to people who cannot afford to pay for it through other social support measures.[11] In so doing, the community has expressed, in part, its moral obligations to the indigent. It seems clear that a similar case can be advanced with respect to community responsibility for health care.

However, since the cost of medical education is supplemented through public funds, physicians have an inherent obligation to offer some of their time in order to provide services to the community on a *pro bono* basis. Some commentators have suggested that only individual physicians have such obligations rather than their employing entities. However, in the case of for-profit plans, it is clear that these organizations and their shareholders are beneficiaries of publicly-supported physician training.[12] Thus, for-profit managed care organizations should play a significant role in the financial support of the *pro bono* work of their physician employees. Beyond these requirements, however, for-profit managed care organizations do not necessarily have moral duties to dispense care without remuneration. This is not to suggest, however, that these organizations do not have other significant moral obligations to their surrounding communities. A number of these obligations will be described in the final chapter.

Even if society could make arrangements so that health care was somehow given away without recompense, there is some question as to whether or not this might be the most socially desirable state of affairs under conditions of fiscal scarcity. From an economic perspective, there is typically little incentive to use "free" goods judiciously. Our recent history under fee-for-service, in which medicine was "free" to many patients because third parties paid the costs with little question, gives evidence of tremendous waste in health care. The Rand Corporation studies cited in chapter 3, which found that the use of health care significantly decreases with cost sharing, gives evidence that "free" goods result in greater waste.[13] Consequently, in the absence of an unlimited pool of resources, there will be even more serious problems of wasteful care and escalating costs in the future, for those who ultimately bear the financial burden.

Next, the assumption that distributing health care exclusively through non-profit organizations is a superior reflection of community morality deserves scrutiny. Since non-profits as well as for-profits have administrative costs, the potential to act competitively, and limited capacities to give away care, the notion that the distribution of care through non-profit organizations alone somehow reflects high societal norms seems dubious.

Some advocates of the exclusive use of non-profits argue that the very concept of earning a profit on medicine is morally suspect because these resources could be poured back into the health care system.[14] While this perspective is also morally appealing, earning a profit on medicine does not overturn an older ethic of service. As stated earlier, medicine has historically involved someone's financial gain. Uwe Reinhardt has pointed out that physicians have always had significant returns on their investment through three main sources of income: a rate of return on remuneration for hours worked; a rate of return on the investment in fixed facilities (the practice); a rate of return on the investment the physician has made in his or her own training. He notes that research has shown that the latter rate is on par with the rate of return to shareholders' equity in other industries.[15]

Given these facts, it seems inconsistent to state that it is acceptable for physicians to earn handsome rates of return on their investment, but it is not acceptable for non-M.D.'s who have invested their savings in the "the mortar and brick" of health care facilities to earn a profit.[16] Despite implications to the contrary, shareholders are not the only ones who benefit from the greater efficiencies these organizations have been able to achieve. Employers, the government, and the broader society have also reaped huge benefits from slower rates of increase in aggregate health care costs.[17] Since shareholders place their capital at risk and add value in the process, it seems reasonable to conclude that they should earn a fair return on their investment.

In the absence of financial incentives, capital is much more difficult to raise, which is perhaps the most critical *disadvantage* of the exclusive use of non-profit plans, a fact even one of their biggest advocates, Arnold Relman, acknowledges.[18] Since non-profit organizations cannot raise funds on the open market, these organizations must rely on debt or internally generated sources of funding through "surpluses" in order to finance capital expansion. Undoubtedly, this can stifle innovation, the ability to keep pace with expensive advances in technology and research, and the hiring of talented employees. Thus, while profit in health care may not be morally ideal, rendering all managed care organizations as *not-for-profit* would eliminate some of the possible efficiency gains which have been created by their growth.

Finally, the idea that the community benefits from the purely symbolic worth of delivery through non-profit managed care organizations seems equally questionable. Medicine as a form of community service had, in years past, much greater meaning with respect to non-profit hospitals, when the stated mission of service to the poor was known to many providers and patients. However, such value seems to be greatly limited in the realm of managed care. The tax-status distinction between the two types of organizations is not (justifiably) very visible in the broader society. In several legal cases, courts have not made a distinction between the two models in overturning denials of benefits to patients. In their rulings, these courts have noted the conflict of the profit motive and fiduciary obligations to patients in non-profit models.[19] Furthermore, it seems that many patients and purchasers in society do not know which organizations are for-profit and which are not. Evidence of this lack of clarity can be seen from the frequent accusations of corporate "greed" which are levied against non-profit organizations.

DIFFERENCES IN ACCOUNTABILITY

Nudelman and Andrews argue that "whereas for-profit organizations are accountable to their shareholders, not-for-profit organizations have another kind of accountability—to patients, to providers of care, to payers, and to the communities in which they operate."[20] Upon a closer examination, it becomes evident that there are several faulty assumptions at work within this claim. First of all, it relies upon the premise that business entities such as for-profit managed care organizations are accountable only to shareholder financial interests. Once again, such a view is based upon the assumption that markets are at best amoral; the "business ethic" is equated with the "custodian of wealth" model of corporate social responsibility. This conception is flawed on both descriptive and normative grounds. Contrary to this understanding of the market, a longer-term view reveals that business organizations are definitely subject to a host of social and ethical constraints on their activities and are not free to restructure an industry in any way they see fit. In addition, there are alternative *normative* models of business that conceive of the aims of for-profit organizations in much broader terms. These more enlightened models, which will be discussed at length in chapter 8, provide a lens through which it can be seen that organizations do not have to be chartered as not-for-profit to serve important moral ends.

However, even if it is granted that the "custodian of wealth" model is accurate from a descriptive standpoint, and that managers of corporations are exclusively bound as fiduciaries to maximize shareholder wealth, there are still limits on an organization's power to reshape the health care environment. In addition to the market-driven changes which may favor patients, discussed earlier, there are other examples of this dynamic in a health care environment.[21] Norman Daniels points out that administrators of for-profit health care organizations may recognize that in order to earn financial gains, they must advocate quality and cultivate a reputation for caring about patients. With this goal in mind, they may hire employees who are not directly concerned about profits at all, and whose primary aims are to deliver quality care.[22] In so doing, perhaps even through inadvertence on the part of the employees, profits may actually increase because the quality of care is high and the reputation of the organization is enhanced as a result. Along similar lines, Philip Boyle states that the construct pitting patient interests against those of the organization is a false dichotomy. While acknowledging that the relationship is imperfect, he argues that when patient interests are protected, the institution is being protected as a matter of course.[23]

Accompanying these mistaken beliefs about profit-seeking corporations is a highly exaggerated view of the altruistic motives of non-profits, particularly, the premise that these organizations are solely accountable to patients. Even the previously cited statement by Nudelman and Andrews, that "not-for-profit organizations have another kind of accountability," names several parties that may place conflicting priorities on these organizations. Providers, payers, and communities may all make claims that rival the interests of patients, severely weakening the possibility that the patient-centered ideal can be achieved. On a related note, Brock and Buchanan point out that administrators of non-profit organizations are also accountable to the preferences of board members, which may or may not be in the best interests of patients.[24]

Substantial evidence was presented in chapter 4 that the "medical ethic" is more myth than reality. However, even if a golden age for medicine existed, the argument that non-profits more closely represent the ideal patient-centered ethic demands further investigation. Claims of the superiority of non-profit organizations seem to imply that they can operate without concern for economic matters such as budgets and salaries. Yet, non-profit organizations must pay careful attention to revenues in order to continue to offer their services. Like profit-seeking models, they cannot operate at deficit levels for a long period of time. Non-profit models also earn "profits" in the form of "surpluses" retained when revenues exceed expenses, though these amounts are not distributed to shareholders. It is necessary that non-profit organizations earn these extra amounts in order to finance future maintenance and to fund expansion plans, which include capital improvements and outlays for new technology and research.

Another implication of the belief that non-profit organizations are free from financial constraints is that they can provide almost limitless amounts of care to plan enrollees. Several commentators have stated that non-profits do not face as many of the ethical challenges involving cost tradeoffs as their profit-seeking counterparts. For example, Nudelman and Andrews claim that unlike for-profit entities, their organization does "not dictate or implement insurance-oriented or finance-based restrictions on care or length of hospital stays."[25] It may well be the case that they can avoid these specific cost constraints. However, it is difficult to comprehend how these organizations can continue to offer competitively priced plans and to remain solvent in the absence of some economically related considerations.

DIFFERENCES IN MOTIVES

Assumptions about differences in accountability between for-profit and non-profit plans are accompanied by a host of other, overstated claims about the differences in the underlying motives of the agents of these organizations. The contention is that non-profits are motivated by service, while shareholder-owned plans are motivated by profit.

The proponents of such claims seem to take for granted the idea that the tax status of organizations will determine the motives of their employees. In particular, they assume that the motives of the employees of non-profit organizations will be altruistic whereas those of profit-seeking ones will be self-interested, resulting in comparatively less consideration of the medical needs of patients. Yet, in addition to the courts who have overlooked the distinction, several commentators have observed that some organizations that are "legally not-for-profit are motivated primarily by concern for margin and market share."[26]

Daniels has pointed out that it is erroneous to believe that the legal charter of the organization alone can determine motives. He states that the "motives of agents within an institution vary depending upon their institutional roles, not on the legal charter of the institution."[27] He argues further that even if upper-level managers of a for-profit organization have the maximization of profit as their primary goal, physicians working within these organizations might be insulated from concerns over the institutional bottom line. As a result, they might not be concerned with the goal of profit at all. Conversely, physicians employed by a non-profit institution may be remunerated according to capitation arrangements or other payment systems rewarding them for containing costs. Consequently, these physicians may be guided by the profit motive, though their employing organization is technically chartered as not-for-profit.[28]

Given the entrepreneurial ethos of medicine that American physicians have practiced under other payment arrangements and the current downward pressure on physician incomes, it seems certain that the potential for being motivated by financial gain will continue to exist. This would be the case even if all managed care organizations were chartered as non-profit and run by physician-owned groups. Indeed, there is evidence suggesting that when doctors are asked to control their own utilization in network-model HMOs, they have used many tools which are similar to those employed by insurers.[29]

Furthermore, since non-profits must make future financial plans, it is likely that administrators of these organizations approach decisions regarding financial matters in a manner indistinguishable from that of executives of their for-profit counterparts. It is also likely that motives and actual employee behavior are determined to a large extent by factors such as internal politics and career goals. These influences are significant regardless of the tax-status of the organization.

DIFFERENCES IN BEHAVIOR

Along with these presumed differences in accountability and motives, Non-Profit Organization Supporters believe that the stated purposes of the two type of organizations will translate into significant *behavioral* differences. Thus, it is critical to examine whether or not non-profits actually act in ways in which overall quality and access to medical care by the poor are improved.

Cases in which non-profit organizations like Kaiser have been involved in controversial cost-cutting practices have made headlines. Overall, the available evidence, though limited, suggests that behavioral differences between the two models are not significant.[30] Since both types of organizations must carry out similar tasks and operate within the same economic climate, this is to be expected. However, claims to the opposite effect persist.

For instance, some observers state that non-profits exclusively are interested in the improvement of quality through developing treatment improvement data, offering preventative care, implementing educational programs for patients and doctors, and providing research opportunities.[31] However, no proof is offered to support this claim. Furthermore, this statement overlooks the fact that for-profit organizations have incentives to engage in similar practices, since their neglect can result in significantly reduced abilities to compete for enrollees and can lead to greater costs in the longer term. In fact, quality improvement programs implemented by for-profit organizations have been heralded as models by researchers in several instances.[32]

In terms of the specific criteria of accessibility, some observers have noted that for-profit managed care organizations "cherry pick" because their publicity campaigns are not targeted to patients with illnesses that are costly to treat, such as HIV infection. Despite inconclusive evidence, it has been further claimed that "financially savvy HMOs" do not focus on preventative care because it is costly in the short run and because most of the long-term savings will accrue to future insurers, due to high turnover rates among plan enrollees.[33] While these are serious concerns that must be addressed, their application extends beyond the scope of for-profit plans. Once again, the observation can be made that unless they possess unlimited resources, non-profit plans must also be conscious of expense and can not afford to eagerly sign up patients with HIV or other costly conditions. Assuming the truth of these accusations, it stands to reason that non-profits have similar incentives to avoid expenditures on preventative care, since these organizations also experience high turnover rates.

Advocates of non-profit organizations also cite differences in various statistical measures as evidence of the behavioral superiority of their model. Comparisons in both the popular and scholarly literature frequently point out large discrepancies in the amounts the two models allocate directly to medical care versus administrative costs and profits. These allocations are commonly measured by medical-loss ratios (MLRs).[34] Typically, observers have noted that non-profits have much higher ratios, indicating that they are spending more on health care. Since premiums are set by market forces, and the actual costs of the plans tend to be very close due to competition, the common conclusion is that for-profits must be reducing the amount they spend on doctors, tests, treatments, and hospitalizations in order to improve their bottom line.[35]

If these ratios are accurate indices of actual qualitative differences between the two models, they would offer much assistance to consumers and personnel managers who are in the process of selecting plans. After all, it would seem to make good sense to enroll in plans that directly spend the most on medical care versus operational expenses and profit distributions. However, when these figures are cited to support the case against for-profit plans, the differences between the models are often overstated, misleading the public in the process. For example, some prominent critics of managed care organizations have been quoted as saying that "for-profit groups skim off 20–30% of premiums as profits before paying for care."[36] Other observers claim that while the 30 percent in question represents the total amount of administrative costs, it includes "extraordinarily large CEO salaries and bonuses, dividends to shareholders, and cash reserves for acquisition of competitors."[37] These numbers are usually contrasted with the figures of non-profit plans such as Kaiser, whose non-medical costs have been reported at just over 3 percent of income, placing its medical-loss ratio at close to 97 percent.[38]

Data from California, the state in which managed care has made its greatest inroads, suggests that the adequacy of these ratios for comparative purposes is questionable. A review of the actual figures reported to the California Department of Corporations, and made publicly available by a frequently cited yearly report from the California Medical Association (CMA), reveals that some of these comparisons have been made from inaccurate, cursory examinations of the data.[39] For example, no plan reported a figure anywhere close to 20 or 30 percent in profits. The highest reported figure for the years 1992–95 was by Aetna Health Plans of California, Inc., which reported a profit of 13 percent in 1994. By comparison, one non-profit plan reported a profit (surplus) of 9.9 percent during the same period.[40] Furthermore, for-profit plans with enrollments of over 20,000 reported an average profit as a percentage of revenue of only 4.6 percent for 1994, compared to 2.9 percent for non-profit plans.[41] In 1995, according to the yearly CMA report, these figures fell to 3.0 percent for the for-profit plans and 2.1 percent for the non-profit plans, a much smaller difference than what is popularly believed.[42]

While several for-profit plans reported combined administrative costs and profit that totaled in the 20 to 30 percent range, so did some non-profit plans.[43] When compared on an overall basis, non-profit institutions reported that higher percentages of their revenues were spent directly on health care. However, when examined on an individual basis, there were many plans offered by for-profit organizations that outspent non-profit plans directly on health care.[44] In fact, several for-profits were listed among the plans with the ten *highest* medical-loss ratios, including two of the top three. Conversely, several non-profits made the list of those organizations with the *lowest* ratios, including two of the top, or more accurately, bottom three.[45] Thus, while there is a *tendency* for non-profits as a group to outspend their counterparts on health care, tax-status is not the sole determinant of allocations.

Studies such as these often suffer from inconsistencies and other methodological weaknesses which reduce the validity of their conclusions. For example, the introductory comments in the 1995–96 edition of the CMA report states that previous editions failed to account for the taxes paid by for-profits. Instead of net income, the organizations were compared on the basis of gross income, thereby over-inflating the profit figures of for-profit plans.[46] While the amount of taxes paid by for-profits is acknowledged in a footnote, pretax profits are still used as the basis of comparison in the 1995–96 version of the report. This edition also acknowledges that there is a current lack of standardized reporting categories for expenditures, further limiting the comparative value of the studies.[47] In addition to allowing for reductions of profits through taxes, it is also important to recognize that many for-profit organizations do not "distribute" profits to shareholders at all, but rather retain them for long-term organizational needs. This runs contrary to common beliefs about one of the key differences between the two models.

Another possible shortcoming of these types of studies is that they do not account for specific structural differences among delivery models. For example, Kaiser operates under a "staff" model, owning its facilities and directly employing its own physicians. By contrast, some of the other organizations, of both non-profit and for-profit status, operate under models such as IPAs (Independent Practice Associations), in which there are broader networks of facilities and physicians to manage. While the latter model benefits patients because of the availability of more choices, there are clear administrative cost differences. Thus, a more accurate comparison of plans should probably account for these distinctions.

However, even if it is assumed that there is reliable comparative value in these figures and that real differences in medical-loss ratios do exist, caution must be exercised in making inferences regarding quality of care. The line of thinking that "spending more is better" in health care has been one of the main contributory factors to our current fiscal crisis. As noted earlier, several studies have shown that greater financial outlays do not always translate into higher quality of care. Wasteful spending on procedures of dubious clinical value has been a common practice in the past, sometimes harming patients and hurting society by driving up aggregate costs in the process.[48] Thus, the fact that for-profits may spend fewer overall resources on doctors, tests, treatments, and hospitalizations, is not necessarily an indicator that quality is impaired in the process.[49]

In addition to MLRs, another commonly cited set of figures for comparative purposes are surveys of enrollees measuring their overall satisfaction with their plans. Using some of these surveys, several observers have noted that enrollees in non-profits report significantly higher levels of satisfaction than those enrolled in for-profit plans. However, one recent survey of nearly 40,000 Californians who were HMO members and who were either employees or retirees of nine large companies of the Pacific Business Group on Health did not support such a conclusion. The results revealed that enrollees in two small non-profit plans reported higher overall satisfaction rates than members of both large for-profit and non-profit plans. Heading the list were Health Plan of the Redwoods and Lifeguard, two Northern California–based non-profit HMOs. However, FHP/TakeCare and Foundation Health, two large for-profit plans, followed close behind in third and fourth place, ahead of Kaiser. Most striking is the fact that Blue Shield, a non-profit plan, was at the bottom of the list, receiving an overall grade of "C" from those surveyed.[50] Thus, factors other than profit status may play a significant role in patient satisfaction.

These examples provide evidence that a deeper examination of often-cited statistical data show that there is much more to the picture than can be readily gleaned through a cursory comparison of medical-loss ratios and reported satisfaction rates. Differences in spending, satisfaction rates, and quality may be due to factors other than the tax-status of the organizations.

Supporters of non-profits often accuse their profit-seeking counterparts of not properly meeting their moral obligations to serve
the poor. For example, Nudelman and Andrews claim that in contrast to for-profit models whose focus is on return on investment,
non-profit organizations have "the inherent motivation and deep
obligation to produce a different kind of return," including "services to the poor."[51] However, there is no evidence that such services are actually provided in amounts greater than those that
for-profit plans deliver, or on a level which would justify the tax-
exempt status of non-profits.

Similar arguments were advanced in support of non-profit entities in the last decade, during the debate over the profit status
of hospitals. On that matter, Brock and Buchanan found no significant differences in the amount of indigent care provided by
corporate-owned and non-profit hospitals. To be sure, true "public" hospitals did provide much more care for the poor than both
investor-owned and non-profit institutions.[52]

Although there is no data available comparing managed care
plans on this measure, there is reason to conclude that the actual
differences are similar in scope to those of different types of hospitals, and are not great, if they exist at all. Non-profit managed
care organizations are not the equivalent of public hospitals,
which are chartered by law to provide indigent care. Moreover, as
stated earlier, both types of managed care organizations may have
conflicting motives at various levels of their hierarchies. Even if
the actual "motivation" to serve the poor is present, economic reality may dictate that less than the desired amount of such care
can be offered. While providing for indigent care is an important
social policy matter, we as a society should move away from the
false belief that non-profits are solely motivated by altruistic concerns and unlimited resources to meet these needs.

Profit-seeking managed care organizations are also accused
of harming poorer members of society by "cream skimming,"
through restricting the process of cost-shifting. Several responses
can be offered to counter this claim. First, "cream skimming" is
not a new practice introduced by the cost-reduction initiatives of

managed care organizations. Independent physicians have always skimmed the "economic cream" to some degree. As mentioned earlier, this is permitted by their code of ethics, which states that they can deny treatment to whomever they please, including those who cannot pay.[53] Second, it is not clear that non-profit managed care plans engage in any less "skimming," given that they too must limit expenses. Finally, while providing for the poor is critical, there are more democratic ways to achieve this than by the hidden process of charging more to those who can pay in order to cover the costs of treating those who cannot.

The evidence from a comparison of the two models suggests that we should avoid pinning false hopes on the exclusive use of non-profit organizations as a comprehensive solution to morally controversial practices in the delivery of managed health care. I am not suggesting that because the two models are more similar than a casual examination would indicate, society should simply accept the dominance of shareholder-owned models without further question. Such a suggestion would commit the naturalistic fallacy—it would fail to address the normative question of what ought to be the case. In light of the previous examples, however, the belief that the path to the service ideal is through the exclusive use of non-profit organizations fails to stand up under scrutiny. The only possible way to facilitate an ideal "social service" model of medicine may be through a thoroughly non-competitive financing and delivery system. Such a system would have to be governmentally controlled, much like the Swedish model. Furthermore, in order to remain consistent with the implications of "service" and to eradicate the possibility of "profiting" on health care, the system would need to be even more radical. Physicians would have to be paid as social servants and would not be allowed to compete with each other over the prospect of greater financial gain. Clearly, the political feasibility of such a system in the United States is very much in doubt. However, even if such a system gained popular acceptance and were implemented, it is certain that at some point, a draconian form of rationing would have to be implemented unless society decided to infinitely fund all claims to health care.[54] It is difficult to imagine how such a model would generate adequate funding, encourage innovation and efficiency, or compete financially in order to attract talented members of society to the profession. As Reinhardt states it, whether we like it or not, medicine is an industry that is far too complex to be run by "missionaries and candy stripers" and, therefore, it must pay wages competitive with other industries in order to attract talented professionals.[55]

Seven   The Moral Viability of For-Profit Organizations

The differences between non-profit and for-profit managed care organizations are not as great as what many people believe. This can be clearly seen when the two models are systematically compared on a number of important dimensions. Their tax status alone is an inadequate indicator of the morality of these organizations.

One possible conclusion is that the non-profit and for-profit distinction is a matter of indifference; both types of organizations are subject to the same forces, and may act morally or immorally, and efficiently or inefficiently. In contrast, those earlier identified as "For-Profit Managed Care Champions" argue that profit-seeking models are *superior* and should be encouraged, because they are better able to meet the demand for more cost-efficient medicine. Malik Hasan, chairman of the shareholder-owned Health Systems International, the parent company of Health Net, has argued that non-profits "are not well suited to the current environment and should be eliminated."[1]

Difficult questions arise with respect to statements about the superiority of either model. We have already seen in the last chapter that freedom from the obligation to return wealth to shareholders will not necessarily lead to better service for patients. The converse argument is that market competition, driven by an undisguised profit motive, is the best means to encourage improved quality and efficiency. After all, it is consistent with principles applied in the market for other goods and services.

AN ETHICAL CRITIQUE OF THE ARGUMENTS OF FOR-PROFIT MANAGED CARE CHAMPIONS

For-Profit Managed Care Champions argue that the accountability created by the profit motive and marketplace competition provides the only means whereby efficiency will be increased, quality improved, and prices lowered for the consumer.[2] Similar to the functioning of the economy for other goods, market discipline will force organizations to improve in all of these areas if they want to successfully compete for a share of the available consumer dollars. Plans that fail to cut waste or to offer quality products and services at competitive prices will soon find themselves without enrollees.

Consistent with a neo-classical economic understanding of the operations of the marketplace, these advocates argue that there should be as little regulatory influence on health care exchanges as possible. By allowing the market to operate with only the minimum restrictions necessary to prevent fraud and enforce contracts, the greatest overall amount of efficiency can be achieved. As a result, many of the proponents of this viewpoint tend to oppose greater regulations on the practices of managed care organizations.[3]

For-Profit Managed Care Champions argue further that investor-owned organizations offer the best model to operate within a competitive marketplace from an efficiency standpoint. Since the profit motive makes managers of these organizations directly accountable to consumers and shareholders, they claim that "investor owned plans are more creative, more aggressive, and more responsive to the demands of service, quality, and affordability."[4] While not all who take this position state they would like to see the elimination of non-profit entities, Hasan has gone as far as to declare that non-profits are financially and organizationally structured in such a way that they cannot compete in the current environment. He states that their survival in past years was due to a lack of true competition for patients, and that non-profit organizations, through their tax exemptions, siphon off sources of government funds that could be used to enact important legislative reforms. Therefore, he argues that such models should either be eliminated or forced to convert to for-profit status in order to compete on equal grounds and pay their fair share of taxes.[5]

Supporters of for-profit organizations cite the explosive growth of enrollees in plans offered by profit-seeking organizations during the last decade and the relatively high satisfaction rates among patients as proof that these organizations are indeed meeting marketplace demands by providing better products at lower prices.[6] Moreover, they assert that in the absence of the growth of profit-seeking plans, there would be much more waste and inefficiency in health care. Gains in efficiency have been made because nonprofits have also been forced to increase their level of operational efficiency in order to compete with for-profit plans.[7]

In response to accusations that shareholder-owned models are incapable of serving patient needs because of the inherent conflict of the profit motive and the healing mission, advocates of profit-seeking organizations respond that many of these concerns are overstated. They claim that the goal of profit and the aim of patient health are not contradictory endeavors. In fact, they argue that the opposite is true because the market makes it in the best interest of for-profit plans to keep enrollees well in the first place; the poor health of patients will cost them more later.[8] Thus, profits are being made on the maintenance of good health. The financial incentives created by the market mandate that their activities are focused on prevention and wellness rather than on withholding necessary procedures.[9] One example of the market's power, as one observer points out, is that in some situations, managed care programs offer mental health benefits which go beyond federal- and state-mandated benefits packages.[10] Furthermore, supporters claim that necessary care is not withheld; the available outcomes data indicate that managed care plans do not reduce the utilization of services.[11]

Some supporters of the profit motive in medicine also argue from the perspective of economic liberty and the freedom to contract. For example, Engelhardt and Rie claim that for-profit medicine in general is "ethical" because it is a product of the free choice of consenting adults.[12] Furthermore, Mark Waymack has argued that some of the most morally troubling aspects of managed care, such as cost-containment measures and coverage restrictions, are not ethical problems because patients have willingly expressed their choices as economic actors. In so doing, they have freely made the tradeoff by contracting for fewer services in exchange for monetary savings. Therefore, they cannot rightfully blame their insurer when specific procedures are not covered.[13]

These arguments, while intuitively appealing to the desire for greater efficiency and the value of freedom, have some major weaknesses. I have claimed that the market has *some* power to regulate the actors and has done so to some degree already. In considering their own long-term interests, organizations do have incentives to behave in accordance with surrounding cultural norms, even under a *laissez-faire* economic model. However, the power of the marketplace to adequately enforce behavior is limited to situations in which consumers have access to high levels of information and bargaining power. Utilizing these criteria, it can be seen that the level at which managed care organizations are governed, given the current lack of regulatory reforms, is nowhere near the point where patient interests are sufficiently protected.

As I stated earlier, it is difficult for consumers to simply vote with their dollars and enroll in other plans if their current organization withholds care or engages in other unethical practices. While a free-market model may work efficiently to regulate the behavior of suppliers of other consumer goods, medicine is clearly subject to "market failure" without some significant provisions for a more level playing field.

The arguments cited above from economic liberty fail to recognize that there are marked differences between medicine and the market for other goods. Such claims falsely assume that a "contract" model is adequate to govern economic exchanges in health care. As discussed in the earlier assessment of Medical Savings Accounts, most patients do not possess the knowledge and skills necessary to act as "lay doctors" and serve as watchdogs over their providers. It is extremely difficult for most patients to recognize appropriate amounts of care and the quality of the services they have received. Even if an adequate level of knowledge were attainable, most patients seek care under conditions of illness and cannot comparison-shop for needed services, placing them at a tremendous disadvantage. Furthermore, in response to Waymack's assertions, patients cannot reasonably anticipate their health care needs sufficiently to "contract" adequately for every possible service prior to having a need for them. The fact is that patients are not equal parties to the relationship with respect to purchasing health care. While more individual responsibility should be encouraged in medical arrangements in the current climate of fiscal limits, our legal tradition has correctly recognized that we cannot reasonably expect patients to possess information on a par with providers or insurers in the broader health care environment.

For a number of reasons, this dynamic holds true within specific managed care settings. First, the end consumers are often not the purchasers, since employers pay for most managed care plans. While a growing number of employers are taking their workers' interests to heart by joining coalitions to accredit managed care plans, there are still others whose sole interest is to find the least costly option. Secondly, many employers greatly limit the choices of plans available to their employees. While the numbers are in dispute, some surveys show that as many as 45 percent of employers offer only one choice of insurance plans to their employees.[14] The numbers are even more discouraging among employers with less than fifty workers. One survey reported that 86 percent offer only one plan.[15] Some employers offer a fee-for-service plan, but a growing number furnish managed care plans with limited provider choices.[16] Thus, the presumed power of choice and the ability of patients to vote with their dollars is quite limited.

Even if the purchasers and the end users of managed care were identical or their interests were perfectly aligned, the current lack of uniform regulations exacerbates the problem of asymmetrical power and the unavailability of the "perfect information" necessary for consumers to regulate unscrupulous actors. This is clearly the case given the lack of legal remedies available because of the ERISA loophole (described in chapter 1), and given the lack of uniform guidelines regulating practices such as the disclosure of physician remuneration arrangements or non-covered treatment options.[17]

Another weakness of some of the arguments used in support of for-profit models is that efficiency is the sole guideline for weighing reform options. While greater efficiency should be one of the goals of major changes in the health care system, the morality of the means to achieve these advancements must also be considered. Significant non-financial costs can be ignored in the quest for aggregate-level efficiencies. For example, the extensive use of non-covered treatment clauses, gag orders, and early release policies may be able to create some short-term efficiencies at the direct expense of moral obligations to improve patient health.

More importantly, the very notion that the greatest efficiencies can be created with the least restrained marketplace might well be flawed. While this will be addressed in greater detail in the next chapter, it certainly seems to go against the conclusions of Adam Smith, the founder of classical economics. Smith held that the greatest economic efficiency was created through equally matched parties.[18]

Also questionable is the contention that there is little need for regulations: the profit motive goes hand-in-hand with the healing mission because of the efficiencies created by preventative care. Clearly, there are instances in which long-term profits clash with the healing mission. For example, without some external guarantee of fairness in sharing the burden, there would be no incentive to be the first plan to pay for expensive new treatments, even those of proven efficacy. This would especially be the case for those treatments in which the costs exceed the benefits, as measured by revenue from new subscribers attracted to the plan as a result of offered coverage.[19] In fact, one Health Net executive stated openly, with respect to cutting-edge cancer research, in the case involving Christy deMeurers, "I can't pay for it if my competitors won't pay for it."[20]

The market actually provides incentives to skimp on preventative care, since there are such high annual disenrollment figures due to personal choice, individual employment changes, or employer plan changes.[21] Without some provisions for portability, and a non-preexisting condition clause which would assure that each managed care organization has a fair share of patients with more serious illnesses, preventative outlays of one plan may serve to benefit another plan.

Finally, it is also an erroneous argument that for-profits should be exclusively used because non-profit entities are less responsive to consumer demands, since they are not accountable to market discipline. As I have noted earlier, though non-profit plans might be at a significant disadvantage in raising capital, there is scant evidence to support the claim that there are significant differences in the accountability and behavior of the two types of models. Patients should be free to make choices between plans offered by both.

Taken together, the arguments of the last chapter and the present one point to the conclusion that both for-profit and non-profit models are viable for health care delivery. However, given their similarities, both have the potential to engage in activities that harm patients. Thus, both are in need of a moral framework that binds them to serve patient and societal interests.

A CASE FOR CAUTIOUS SUPPORT OF MANAGED CARE

The emergence of managed care and the subsequent growth in market competition has resulted in vast improvements in aggregate-level efficiency. The long-held monopolistic power of physicians to set prices and artificially create demand for unnecessary procedures and services has been broken. Premium rates have stabilized and in some situations have actually decreased.[22]

Much to the dismay of organized medicine, competition and the use of selective contracting are forcing reductions in capacity. This has directly resulted in savings through closures of unnecessary facilities, a reduction in the demand for expensive and unnecessary specialist procedures, and falling physician incomes.[23] For example, until recently, 40 percent of hospital beds were empty on an average day, resulting in costly excess capacity.[24] Prior to the growth of managed care, there was a rapid increase in the number of specialists. This resulted in an increase in the number of specialty procedures being performed in order to keep incomes high. Managed care has acted to reduce both extra capacity and the number of specialists to a point now where they more accurately reflect true market demand.[25] In achieving these economic efficiencies, costs have been stabilized and access should thereby improve.

Although there is very real potential for gaining efficiencies at the expense of quality care, the market model does hold some promise in regulating behavior and encouraging quality improvements. In fact, some shareholder-owned organizations have model quality measures and monitoring systems to ensure that doctors are not skimping on needed care, including preventative care.[26] For example, U.S. HealthCare has a catastrophic illness adjustment for doctors who have sicker-than-average patient loads. In addition, physicians who work for this organization are free to discuss their compensation model, which has been published, with patients.[27] Furthermore, as noted earlier, several studies have indicated that on the whole, patients enrolled in health maintenance organization models have better access to preventative measures than those in fee-for-service plans.

There is some evidence that the current profit margins that have raised so much public concern are already beginning to decrease.[28] Some observers predict that as price competition continues and margins fall, the basis of competition will shift directly to quality, leading to even greater improvement in care.[29] Some organizations are already using such programs to differentiate themselves from the competition. For example, Blue Shield recently announced that it would allow its HMO plan enrollees to bypass gatekeepers and self-refer to specialists for an additional copayment of twenty dollars. Many other plans are expected to follow suit.[30] In addition, triple-option plans have been introduced in response for patient demands for broader access. These plans allow patients to see any doctor or specialist of their choice, even those outside of the network, in exchange for a higher out-of-pocket fee.

While managed care, including the involvement of shareholder-owned plans, is supportable, there are good reasons to fear that some of the prevalent practices will lead to grave patient and societal harm. Given the similarities between for-profits and non-profits, the latter are not immune from the potential for unethical behavior by virtue of their tax-exempt status. Thus, while the employment of for-profit organizations is acceptable, some of the practices of both models are not. Managed care has the most promise of any of the reform measures, but the organizations involved in its delivery need to be grounded in an ethic that properly guides their behavior. A restrained marketplace is necessary to protect the rights of all parties, above all the patients. Managed care organizations, regardless of tax status, must be governed by an ethical framework which will ensure that they will work towards the norms of justice set forth earlier in this work. Such a framework must address both the business and medical functions of these organizations.

This perspective can be placed under the auspices of the type I have identified as "Cautious Supporters of Managed Care." It is an important intermediary position in this debate, since it advocates the positive aspects of managed care and the role of for-profit organizations within it but acknowledges some critical limits of a free-market approach. My contention is that the Cautious Supporter position is the most morally defensible one. It recognizes the pressing need for a set of ethical norms from which moral responsibilities and social policies can be developed to govern the activities of managed care organizations.

However, developing such ethical norms is problematic. Even a position of *cautious*, as opposed to unreserved, support is attempting to bring together two realms, business and medicine, whose missions apparently follow widely diverging paths. The question is how the two can be integrated effectively. Managed care organizations are in the tenuous position of attempting to function simultaneously as both traditional businesses with obligations to return financial gains to shareholders and to produce profits (or "surpluses"), and as medical providers with duties to uphold the primacy of patient health. Thus, normative standards applicable to one function do not transfer smoothly to the other.

The possibility of developing an ethical paradigm, which accounts for both the business and medical roles of these institutions, seems to some difficult if not altogether impossible. Past attempts at formulating a governing paradigm have fallen short because they have grounded the ethical obligations of these organizations in either traditional medical norms or *laissez-faire* market morality. Wendy Mariner notes that the resulting standards tend to reflect exclusively either the business or medical aspects of these organizations, but not both.[31] She acknowledges that there are times that business corporations can satisfy both shareholders and customers, especially when socially responsible practices are popular and therefore profitable. However, when "an MCO's financial goals conflict with its service methods, little in the field of business ethics argues for giving subscribers priority."[32] Thus, significant questions linger with respect to a governing paradigm for organizations with a foot in both the business and medical camps. Moreover, the ethical discussion so far has been concentrated on the obligations of individual physicians, leaving the formation of ethics for organizations as *organizations* almost undeveloped.[33] The next chapter addresses the question of whether there is sufficient overlap between the realms of business and medicine to formulate guidelines that account for both functions of managed care organizations. On this point hangs the possibility of developing an integrative ethical model for MCOs from which flow moral responsibilities.

Eight Business Ethics for Managed Care Organizations

REASSESSING THE DIFFERENCES
BETWEEN MEDICINE AND BUSINESS

The antithetical portrayal of business and medicine appeals to common perceptions of business organizations and the actors within them as immoral or, at a minimum, amoral.[1] Arguably, much of commerce may be described as taking place in the belief that Adam Smith's "invisible hand" guides the affairs of the marketplace for the common good, so long as parties to economic transactions are free to pursue their own self-interest. Economists of the neo-classical school of thought have done much to advance this notion in their portrayals of the single-minded motivation of *homo economicus*.[2] Milton Friedman, in his often cited essay, "The Social Responsibility of Business Is to Increase Its Profits," has contributed to this perception through his contention that investor rights to maximization of share price should reign supreme.[3]

Such depictions of the commercial marketplace contrast sharply with those of health care, which is usually cast in morally heroic terms of charity and altruism.[4] When the predominantly negative image of business is set against this depiction of medicine, it is no wonder that the emerging dominance of shareholder-owned business organizations in managed care is perceived as an ominous threat to patient and societal well-being.

As pointed out in an earlier chapter, negative sentiments about the involvement of business in medicine rest upon erroneous assumptions of the differences between these two arenas. Andrew Wicks argues that these portrayals fall short due to their very narrow conception of business and the place of morality within it, together with their exaggerated conception of the heroic nature of health care professionals.[5] These are excellent reasons why the perception of antithesis between medicine and business should be rejected, and in its place, a reformulated view should be constructed.[6]

One of the primary reasons to reject such a pessimistic view of business is that business has a rich moral tradition that goes well beyond profit maximization. Patricia Werhane's research reveals that a narrow, egoistic approach to business is a betrayal of Adam Smith's original vision of a free-market economy. Far from advocating a mechanism to simply empower individual acquisitiveness, Smith was much more concerned with creating a commercial system which would serve the common good.

Werhane argues that Smith is commonly misunderstood as advancing the theory that a free, unregulated market, driven by unrestrained self-interest and competition, will function autonomously, like the physical laws of gravity, and automatically will lead to the greatest efficiencies possible. Contrary to this interpretation, she asserts that Smith's *Wealth of Nations* should be understood in conjunction with the moral restraints expressed in his *Theory of Moral Sentiments*. Werhane argues that Smith envisioned a market where the players must exercise self-restraint, since greed *prevents* rather then promotes good economic performance. Instead of postulating total freedom from ethical and legal limits, Smith believed that the market functions as an adequate regulator only to the extent that participants in economic transactions exercise self-restraint and there is fair competition in a climate of judicial enforcement.[7]

This reinterpretation of Adam Smith depends on three critical points, each of which is directly applicable to the development of a moral framework for managed care organizations. The first is that Smith makes an important distinction between self-interest and greed, by noting that avarice serves to impede the proper functioning of the market rather than enhance it.[8] Contrary to popular perception, then, ethics and self-restraint play irreplaceable roles in market transactions. Practical evidence of Smith's idea of the place of morality as an important cornerstone for the economy can be seen in the daily affairs of business.[9] Philip Boyle states that if these values were missing and all business transactions were conducted according to the opposite norms, such as giving inaccurate information or biased recommendations to entice customers to purchase unneeded goods, business would come to a halt.[10]

Second, Smith believed that perfect competition occurs only when both parties to an exchange are equally matched. This is not to imply that he favored equality of outcomes, but rather that the market is most efficient and fair when there is competition between parties who are standing on equal ground.[11] This gives us reason to question, from a business perspective, the fairness of some managed care arrangements, given the current asymmetries in bargaining power between patients, physicians, and insurers. Third, instead of a completely free market with no restraints, there is a legitimate place for a third-party watchdog in efficient markets, especially in situations in which there is a disparity in bargaining power between the parties to a transaction.

Such a rereading of Smith leads to the conclusion that the model of the efficient market as either immoral, or at best amoral, should be rejected. Smith's analysis is far from a defense of a greed-ridden *laissez-faire* description of the marketplace. There is considerable room in Werhane's interpretation of Smith for broad moral standards within business, including those which are promising with respect to transactions involving health care.

Another reason Wicks rejects the antithetical portrayal of business and medicine is that it relies upon an unrealistic view of ethics and human nature. In sharp contrast to Adam Smith's distinction between self-interest and selfishness, common depictions of business (and ethics) fail to distinguish these two motives.[12] The fusion of self-interest with selfishness leads to the narrow view that ethical behavior must be based solely upon altruism. This view relies upon an unrealistic understanding of human behavior, since it assumes that ethical behavior cannot be motivated by any form of self-interest. In opposition, numerous scholars, including Michael Novak, have stated that there can be virtuous forms of self-interest in addition to morally neutral or evil forms of it. For example, Novak cites a person's desire to develop his or her talents, or to develop self-mastery and control, as forms of self-interest which are not evil in nature.[13]

The effacement of the distinction between self-interest and selfishness results in what R. Edward Freeman has termed the "two realms" problem or "the separation thesis," according to which ethics is incompatible with business since the former necessarily rejects self-interest while the latter upholds it.[14] If this were true, the possibility of ethical actions in medicine would also be severely limited. Yet, the "two realms" view is almost exclusively extended to business, while health care professionals are commonly perceived to be primarily interested in the selfless advancement of the well-being of patients.

As discussed in chapter 4, a reexamination of medicine reveals that it has a strong "business" dimension to it. Numerous examples of financially-motivated behavior offer evidence that physicians are not nearly as charitable as they have been portrayed. While we should be clear that there are many physicians (as there are business people) who are motivated by altruistic concerns, these factors should temper the view of medicine as a profession which is devoid of self-interest (and selfishness).

As such, there are good reasons to reject a portrayal of medicine and business in which they are placed on opposite ends of the moral spectrum. However, a reasonable objection could be raised that the use of such egregious examples from the realm of medicine is unfair. One could argue that these examples represent the worst aspects of medicine rather than its prevailing ethos and as such, are a mere distortion of medical norms. In contrast, one could argue, the state of moral normalcy in business is much lower than the prevailing state of affairs in medicine. Or, in other words, *everyday* business activity is comparable in nature to morally suspect *exceptional* behavior in the practice of medicine.

Several responses to these claims are possible. First, in reinterpreting Adam Smith's vision of a free market, unethical business activities can also be seen as mere "distortions" of an ideal. Various forms of commercial behavior can be interpreted in this light, along the lines of recent criticisms of the medical profession. Second, a reexamination of actual commercial practice reveals that "business as usual" cannot be accurately characterized as a profit-at-all-cost game of avarice and deceit.

Accompanying the earlier-mentioned argument that the proper functioning of a market economy presupposes a moral foundation, there is some empirical evidence to suggest that investor expectations do not fit neo-classical economic assumptions of profit maximization. In fact, shareholders often have ethical concerns which temper their desire for profit. For instance, shareholders who have social concerns about the environment may want the firm in which they have hold equity to go beyond legal requirements to minimize pollution, even at a reduction in the price of their shares or dividends. Another example is the reaction of many shareholders to doing business in South Africa under apartheid. While these may seem rare occurrences at best, a recent study by Pietra Rivoli confirms that shareholders do in fact often behave in ways that are other-interested. In her study of voting patterns, she concludes that stockholders, including those who are educated and involved, often violate neo-classical economic assumptions and vote in favor of initiatives which limit profits for the sake of other social goods.[15]

Rivoli's research seems to confirm a more realistic assessment of business and a more complex portrayal of the combination of motives and norms that guide human behavior. Clearly, self-interest is just one element in the equation; human beings can be other-interested in their pursuit of financial gain. In pointing out that "few people are as greedy as Ivan Boesky or as altruistic as Albert Schweitzer," Wicks states that most human behavior takes place "in the realm in-between where there are a variety of motives and where practices have common elements of both self-interest and regard for others."[16]

Rather than accepting the "two realms" conception, it is more accurate to assume that most human actions take place with *some* degree of self-interest at heart. Thus, Smith's observation that there is a tremendous difference between self-interest and selfishness or greed is critical. The former allows room for self-restraint through the consideration of other moral interests, while the latter does not. Wicks states that a more realistic account of human nature acknowledges that self-interest, shaped and tempered by a variety of other moral considerations, does and should play a prominent role in business as it does in medicine and other professions.[17]

A reassessment of business and medicine shows that they are not necessarily antithetical and opens the door to the possibility of developing a moral paradigm for managed care organizations.

However, to state that "business as usual" is not as negative as has been portrayed should not be interpreted as an argument in favor of a *laissez-faire* shareholder maximization model for managed care. I am not arguing that commerce is free from unethical behavior or that the market will somehow always correct itself. This type of approach is clearly inadequate in a health care environment, because scenarios in which financial interests prevail at the expense of patient health would certainly occur. Thankfully, this is not the only model for business activity in theory *and* in actual practice.

CONTRIBUTIONS FROM BUSINESS ETHICS

In the field of business ethics, a host of competing normative paradigms of corporate responsibility have been advanced to counter Friedman's "custodian of wealth" model.[18] One approach in particular, the stakeholder theory, has recently had a profound influence on the direction of business ethics, business and society research, and actual business practice.[19]

Early formulations of the stakeholder theory, as developed by R. Edward Freeman in conjunction with William Evan, expand moral duties to include "multi-fiduciary" reciprocal relationships to stakeholder groups, such as employees, customers, suppliers, and the local community. The theory is based upon a Kantian conception of respect for persons. The corporation, rather than being an instrument which functions solely for wealth maximization, is a vehicle whereby "each stakeholder group makes itself better off through voluntary exchanges."[20] It is important to note that this construct does not jettison the property rights of shareholders. In addition to acknowledging the financial contributions of shareholders to the existence and success of the corporation, however, the model offers extended recognition of the value added by other stakeholders. For example, it acknowledges the contributions of labor and talent from employees and the specific moral obligations owed to these parties as a result. While proponents grant that a perfect harmony can never be achieved, the normative goal of this approach is to strike a balance between the stakes of the competing groups.

Early formulations of the theory are promising with respect to the expansion of corporate social responsibility. However, one of the common criticisms of the approach is that it seems to lack a clear moral foundation, which is essential to resolving conflicts between stakeholder groups.[21] This is in contrast, for instance, to the property rights grounding of the "custodian of wealth" model. However, in more recent formulations, Freeman has stated that the "stakeholder theory" can be expanded into a number of "stakeholder theories," each having a "normative core" that can serve as a set of standards in determining the purposes of corporations and the way managers should carry out their duties.[22]

While Freeman states that there are a number of political theories that could serve as the basis of a normative core, he has developed one conception based upon the notions of autonomy and fairness as articulated by John Rawls and other thinkers from the pragmatic liberal tradition. Within this conception, Freeman notes:

> The normative core for this redesigned contractual theory will capture the liberal idea of fairness if it ensures a basic equality among stakeholders in terms of their moral rights as these are realized in the firm, and if it recognizes that inequalities among stakeholders are justified if they raise the level of the least well-off stakeholder.[23]

The definition of fairness in this context would be driven by Rawls's principles of justice. A contract is fair if parties to it would willingly accept the terms while ignorant of their actual stakes. In other words, as Freeman states it, "a contract is like a fair bet, if each party is willing to turn the tables and accept the other side."[24] In applying this idea to business settings, corporations would be measured against this standard of fairness in stakeholder relationships.

The specific nuances of the stakeholder approach and the possible theories that could serve as the normative core are much too elaborate to discuss in detail here. However, for our purposes, two important points are worth noting. First, stakeholder theory can incorporate Rawlsian principles into a lens through which business conduct can be assessed. Second, various formulations of the model commonly conceive of business in a manner in which it is not only legitimate, but expected, that the "good" is broader than profit maximization.

The stakeholder approach (broadly defined) can be criticized because it appears much too optimistic to serve as an adequate framework for actual marketplace behavior. In addition, the "multi-fiduciary" aspect seems too broad to be operational, given our traditional political-economic and legally based recognition of personal property rights.[25] However, a number of states have adopted "corporate constituency statutes" which at a minimum permit, and at times require, executives to make decisions based upon the impact of corporate actions on non-shareholder constituents. In addition, management scholars see some evidence that business practice is headed toward a direction in which a wider spectrum of moral interests and goals is being incorporated into decision making.[26] In a sense, business is returning to a "unified moral paradigm," similar to that envisioned by Adam Smith.[27] Evidence for this can be seen in the fact that there are a growing number of corporations employing more enlightened business models to guide their daily affairs.

Examples of such practices are prevalent. The well-publicized actions of then seventy-three-year-old Aaron Feuerstein are a good case in point. Giving as a reason his commitment to the community, Feuerstein rebuilt a burned-down manufacturing plant, which was a vital economic lifeline for the town of Muthen, Massachusetts, despite the fact that he could have simply retired on the insurance money. In addition, Feuerstein continued to pay his workers and to provide health care benefits during reconstruction of the facility. Many other corporations which are shareholder-owned, such as Merck, Starbucks, and Johnson and Johnson, function as values-oriented stakeholder enterprises which view their social commitments as being perfectly consistent with their financial success.[28]

Adhering to the description of the complexity of human motivation given earlier, Wicks notes that "altruism" is not a good way to interpret the actions of these corporations.[29] Clearly, these organizations gain financially while engaging in activities benefiting stakeholders. However, such gain does not present a new problem, nor does it describe a dynamic which is only at work in a business setting, since physicians also benefit financially from their services.

The stakeholder approach is a promising one for the new intersections of medicine and business. When specifically applied to managed care arrangements, the model has much more promise to safeguard the interests of patients, physicians, and society at large than the narrow egoistic conception of business.[30] These parties become noteworthy stakeholders whose interests must be considered if an organization is to be judged as behaving ethically. However, several significant challenges still need to be addressed before we can conclude that this theory can adequately account for the dual roles of these organizations.

CHALLENGES TO THE APPLICATION
OF A BUSINESS MODEL TO MEDICINE

A challenge can be raised that under any business-based model, no matter how "enlightened," profit is still a central component of the "good" to which commercial activity aims. Thus, even a restrained pursuit of profit is still at odds with an ethical approach to medicine. For example, Edmund Pellegrino recognizes the distinction between *legitimate* self-interest and selfishness. Yet, he states that "by code or by covenant, the physician promises to serve the interests of the patient, not to exploit the patient or take advantage of the patient's vulnerability. It is the obligation to suppress even legitimate self-interest in this way that characterizes medicine and other professions."[31] Based, in part, upon this view, he is in agreement with numerous others who have argued that profits from health care should be placed back into the system rather than distributed to shareholders.[32] And so he argues for the exclusive use of non-profit organizations.

While non-profit organizations have their place and altruistic behavior should be encouraged, it remains to be seen how the expectation to suppress even legitimate self-interest might be systematized in a workable fashion. As noted earlier, profit in health care has not been newly introduced by managed care organizations. Physicians have earned and continue to earn high incomes.

Consequently, it is quite natural to ask why it is acceptable for doctors to profit from their work, especially when their training is heavily subsidized by the public, while it is not legitimate for investors to earn a reasonable return for their contributions.[33] Shareholders clearly create value by risking their capital for research, expansion, and the acquisition of facilities, equipment, and technology. There are legitimate concerns that returns on investment will to be too large and will thereby subtract too greatly from medical resources. However, the overall amount of profit in managed care has been overstated by critics.[34]

It is also important to remember that non-profit organizations earn profits (known as surpluses) and pay physicians competitive salaries. Additionally, physicians who work for them can still be motivated by self-interest and by selfishness. Consequently, as noted in chapter 6, the only means to consistently eradicate the profit motive in medicine would be to develop a socialized system even more radical than the Swedish model. Doctors would be paid set wages consistent with a social service scale. Although this may have some initial appeal, the ramifications would be profound. It is far from certain that people of the same caliber as those who are currently attracted to medicine would continue to compete so rigorously to engage in its practice.[35] Novak has suggested that a realistic appraisal of complex motives in human behavior demands that we construct an "economy for sinners."[36] While his language may be too strong, his point is well taken. The only workable system is one that adequately accounts for self-interest, especially in the broader sense of the term.

A related challenge which could be raised about the use of a business model is that the specific responsibilities which can be assigned for business functions are insufficient for medical activities. In particular, unlike business, medicine is a profession. Thus, medical practitioners have higher behavioral expectations, such as fiduciary obligations, which are placed upon them by society. Conversely, it is claimed that business is run almost exclusively on a pure contractual model, which extends ethical obligations only to the point of upholding explicitly made promises.[37]

One specific area of conflict stemming from these different expectations can be seen in the disparity over the morally required amount of information disclosure, which is much lower in typical business settings than in medicine. Arnold Reiman notes that unlike physicians, "salesmen and other commercial purveyors" are not ombudsmen for their customers.[38] For example, car dealers are not required to disclose options which they do not include but which their competitors do, while there is a fair amount of agreement that managed care organizations should inform patients of non-covered treatment options. Therefore, some actions that are merely obligatory in medicine would be considered "heroic" in business.

It should be clear by now that these observations rely on familiar, faulty notions of the gap between medicine and business. As a profession, medicine clearly has never been as heroic as it is often portrayed. Fiduciary-level obligations exist only after the patient and physician are in an actual relationship, which the physician has the right to decline to enter into in the first place, nor are such obligations absolute once a relationship is established. In addition, patients have always had to compete for limited resources, because physicians have other patients and their own needs for rest and leisure. Dan Brock further observes that it would be naive to think that by becoming professionals, individuals lose concern for their own interests.[39] It was simply much easier to hide these motives under the older fee-for-service model, since courses of action favoring both the interests of the patient and physician were often identical.

Concomitantly, these observations also rely on the false belief that business runs on a largely amoral contractual model. In addition to growing numbers of corporations which have adopted a more enlightened stakeholder model of behavior, there are a number of participants in business who have traditionally been bound by higher ethical duties. Accountants and architects are examples of "business" people who are regarded as professionals or, at the very least, "quasi-professionals." Because of differences in knowledge, they are held to fiduciary-level obligations to their clients.[40] Although the specific nature and content of these duties may differ from those of physicians, they can be accurately characterized as going beyond a simple contractual model. Thus, there is the possibility of assigning moral responsibilities to organizations and individuals involved in business which go well beyond honoring explicitly rendered agreements.[41]

Furthermore, this more enlightened approach to business has the flexibility of adjusting the level of responsibility according to what is at stake. Unlike the presumed exclusive set of duties to shareholders under the "custodian of wealth" model, stakeholder interests are not a rigid, fixed quantity for all situations. Evan and Freeman state that these interests are not univocal and can vary with industry, organization, and situation.[42] As such, it is appropriate to assign duties to businesses which are synonymous to those which would be held in medicine when similar interests are at stake. For example, in the disclosure example above, a consistent application of the stakeholder approach would require managed care organizations to inform patients of all treatment options whether or not they are covered by the plan. Much more is at risk than whether or not a leather-trim package is available on a particular make of automobile. While no other commercial arrangements may have duties identical to those in medicine, the very fact that managed care organizations are in the business of delivering health care would bind them to unique obligations under the stakeholder model, since context and situation would be relevant considerations in determining responsibilities.

However, even with the possibilities of broader moral considerations under the stakeholder approach, a third significant challenge can be raised with respect to its fit for medicine. The stakeholder model was developed to serve a host of competing interests surrounding a corporation. In contrast, there appears to be only one overriding moral obligation in medicine: to serve the best interest of patients.[43] Thus, the primary ethical principle that has traditionally been assigned to individual physicians does not easily fit with the business aspects of managed care organizations.[44]

While this objection presents a challenge, the point needs to be reiterated that medicine has never met the standard of a completely exclusive focus on the needs of patients. Moreover, fairness mandates that in our current climate of fiscal scarcity, interests other than individual patient needs must be considered. After all, the exclusive focus on individual patients has played a significant role in contributing to our current fiscal crisis.

The fourth possible challenge to extending the stakeholder model comes from the difficulty of assigning ethical obligations to organizations as *organizations*, especially since they have traditionally been regarded as mere "fictitious persons" under the law.[45] This difficulty is amplified in managed care settings, since individual physicians have taken unique oaths to serve patients, while the organizations themselves have not.[46] The troubling question over whether or not organizations are moral agents with concomitant rights and responsibilities has long been a subject of debate among philosophers and, more practically, in the legal system.[47] Within this discussion, the point has been raised that it is only *individuals* within an organization that have moral rights and duties.[48] In addition, the nature and structure of organizations can often diffuse individual ethical responsibility.[49]

While it is difficult, it is not impossible to assign moral responsibilities to organizations. Peter French has argued that because organizations have internal decision-making structures which amount to "corporate intentionality," they qualify as moral agents with reciprocal rights and responsibilities.[50] Thomas Donaldson has stated that corporations, like governments, have moral responsibilities to society in the form of social contracts. These obligations arise because corporations are part and parcel of social systems and networks creating their existence in the first place.[51]

Our legal system acknowledges the fact that actions of organizations can be judged according to normative standards for behavior and that they can be assigned moral responsibilities. For example, organizations will often be penalized for harmful actions brought about by their internal decision-making structures.[52] Furthermore, in bringing legal standards to bear on corporations, Federal Sentencing Guidelines recognize institutional culpability, since they grant *organizations* leniency if internal mechanisms have been in place to prevent illegal actions from occurring.[53] Thus, organizations are often assigned moral responsibilities akin to those of individuals and can therefore be praised or criticized for particular practices.

However, even if it is granted that organizations have moral responsibilities, a fifth concern can be raised with respect to the difficulties inherent in attempting to balance stakeholder interests. In particular, there is no guarantee that patient interests will necessarily be favored when it comes to a direct conflict. Even with respect to more traditional business settings, there is the problem of "stakeholder adjudication," since there is a lack of consensus over how the various interests should be balanced when there is a conflict.[54]

For instance, one stakeholder group may claim that stopping a plant closure in a community is the highest ethical concern because of its potential impact on local employment and company profitability. A rival group may favor closing the plant down because of the pollution or other environmental damage caused by the use of specific materials for the products that the plant is processing. These tensions would only be exacerbated when applied to the realm of medicine, where it would be difficult, if not impossible, to achieve a harmonious balance between the adverse interests of patients, payers, physicians, and societal needs for cost control.

These are valid observations, but they do not negate the value of the stakeholder approach. The contention here is not that a perfect balance can ever be achieved. Rather, my point is to establish the legitimacy of moving towards such a balance by expanding the moral obligations of business organizations from the narrow "custodian of wealth" model. It is also important to note that internal disagreement within the stakeholder approach does not create a new dilemma in its application to health care. There is a clear lack of consensus on important values within the realm of traditional medical ethics as well. For example, continuing disagreements linger over how best to balance autonomy, justice, and benevolence when these priorities conflict in situations of clinical decision making.

Finally, there is some concern that any "business model" will skew the balance towards the interests of the corporation when it comes to a conflict between long-term survival and patient interests, no matter how enlightened the organization. For instance, Mariner expresses worry over whether or not management will have the authority to favor patient interests when they conflict with the financial survival of the organization.[55]

This objection seems fair enough. There is little question that organizational interests will be favored when survival is at stake. However, if conditions ever reach such a drastic state, for-profit organizations would not be the only ones that would tip the balance in favor of financial survival over other stakeholder interests. Individual physician practices, traditional insurance arrangements, non-profits, and even government-run organizations must consider finances at some point and could not continue providing care without limit. Thus, the bias toward organizational survival is not something unique to "business," nor is it a new dimension to medicine.

These significant challenges to the application of a business model to medicine do not negate the value of the approach. The stakeholder approach provides a ready answer to allegations that corporations are solely economic engines for the exclusive purpose of profit maximization. By extending this framework to the realm of managed care, we as a society have much less reason to believe that the solution to ethical problems in medicine must bring with it the eradication of business values. This approach is a great improvement over the traditional narrow conception of business activity, since it legitimates broader moral considerations.

ADVANTAGES OF AN ENLIGHTENED BUSINESS MODEL OVER A TRADITIONAL MEDICAL MODEL

The extension of an enlightened business approach to managed care is a gain over the narrow profit-maximization model. It also has distinct advantages over the traditional charity-based medical model. First, the integration of medicine under an enlightened business model more accurately reflects the realistic picture of human motivation and ethics posited earlier. In lieu of an ethics founded on the concepts of "altruism" and "charity," which leads to the earlier described "two realms" problem, Werhane and Wicks suggest that we should reformulate our view of ethics. Ethics should be founded on concepts such as trust, respect for others, decency, fair play, and justice.[56] These are the appropriate norms to govern interactions between strangers in public and professional life. In addition to being consistent with Rawlsian ethics, concepts such as justice and fair play are also more inclusive of a more complete picture of human beings, because they are less opposed to self-interest, in the correct sense of the term.[57]

A realistic view of ethics and human motivation, then, is not opposed to self-interest but broadens its definition to include a host of other moral considerations. In contrast, the altruism/caring model of ethics leads to the "two realms" problem. As a result, all medical care that is not given away freely can be condemned as unethical since it involves economic gain. Clearly, this conception would label and dismiss almost all actions in medicine which involve financial exchanges as morally inappropriate.

While it would *not* be a challenge to find examples of selfish behavior in both arenas, business and medicine can and often do function according to more enlightened forms of self-interest, which allow for other moral considerations to temper the pursuit of profit. Wicks notes that many physicians serve as prime examples of this dynamic at work. They have been able to serve others without sacrificing their financial well-being.[58] Although service rather than the pursuit of wealth is their stated mission, doctors have traditionally "done well by doing good." The fact that doctors can profit while engaging in service to the community gives us reason to reject the view that business and medicine are essentially incompatible. An enlightened *business* model offers a clear advantage because it allows us to more comprehensively account for the mixed motives at work in the arenas both of business and of medicine.

A second advantage of an enlightened business model is that it allows us to appropriately balance interests in a manner reflecting the current changes in the health care environment. Werhane notes that while caring is a virtue, it is not comprehensive in dealing with health care problems without the underlying virtue of justice, because it does not preclude being arbitrary or unfair to those not included in one's circle of benevolence. Moreover, she points out that charity does not preclude noncooperation or greed.[59] Thus, Rawls's "representative least-advantaged" members of society could suffer great harm. A physician or an organization could provide unlimited care to a select group of patients without consideration of the interests of others. This was clearly the situation under the dominance of the older fee-for-service model of medicine, which contributed to the problem of escalating costs and the placement of health care insurance out of the reach of millions. A stakeholder approach can be formulated so that it values justice (as Rawls defines it) as a central principle in attempting to balance the complex and competing interests that surround particular actions.[60]

Third, a more enlightened understanding of business allows us to consider greater areas of overlap with medicine. This has the practical benefit of moving the debate away from the simplistic "business bashing" that has permeated the current discussion and toward a realistic assignment of moral responsibility. Due in part to the narrow depiction of business, managed care organizations have often been blamed for financially-related treatment decisions which are made by another party, such as an individual physician, a hospital, or a practice group.[61] Workable solutions and policies cannot be developed as long as the wrong party is the target for blame. A more accurate appraisal of business can work towards the development of a more realistic and operational assignment of moral obligations.

Fourth, with our current fiscal crisis, there are other practical advantages to viewing and operating medicine like a business. The consideration of financial limits and the application of business concepts such as total quality management and realignment can undoubtedly improve the efficiency with which medicine is delivered. In turn, scarce resources can be saved and access can be improved for those who have no coverage at all. It is well documented that excess capacity is already being reduced, as the number of physician specialists and empty hospital beds declines.

A fifth advantage is that managed care organizations respond well to norms developed with business-oriented concepts and terms. Although many physicians and the broader public may be uncomfortable with the fact, these institutions are likely to be the dominant model of health care delivery for some time to come. Thus, it is helpful for patients, physicians, and policymakers to be equipped with ideas and concepts from business ethics in order to hold managed care organizations to appropriate levels of moral responsibility.

Finally, as Nancy Jecker insightfully notes, the integration of medicine under a business model brings into sharper focus the various ethical concerns that owning and operating a business entail. These concerns remain hidden as long as medicine is viewed in terms of patient-physician relationships under the caring model, which is mistakenly presumed to be free from a business dimension.[62]

Taken together, these factors offer evidence that an enlightened business model has significant advantages over a traditional medical model, especially when the fiscal constraints of the new health care environment are taken into account. Overall, the stakeholder approach challenges the assumption that corporate business must be conducted for the exclusive purpose of profit maximization. Thus, while it is true that some firms operate on the "greed is good" philosophy, characterizing this as the "business ethic" is both factually inaccurate and logically contradictory. An enlightened approach to business would not support harming patients, in the name of *legitimate* self-interest. The conduct of some managed care organizations around the country does reinforce the notion that they are solely interested in profit at the expense of patient well-being. However, through the lens of a reconceptualized understanding of commercial activity, it is possible to state from a business perspective that these MCOs have been acting unethically in their pursuit of financial gain.

Nine   Stakeholder Responsibilities in the New Health Care Environment

Based upon an enlightened approach to business, numerous moral obligations can be derived for managed care organizations which are consistent with both their medical and business obligations.[1] In light of these responsibilities the growth of managed care plans does not destroy the integrity of medicine.

In addition to the responsibilities of managed care organizations, however, other important stakeholder groups also have reciprocal ethical duties. Specifically, the surrounding community, patients, and employers have distinct obligations. While I have separated these stakeholders for purposes of discussion, they are by nature intimately intertwined. All of these key groups must uphold their responsibilities if health care is to be delivered in an appropriate manner.

It is important to note that the absence of discussion of the ethical duties of individual physicians is not an oversight. Numerous authors have written insightfully on these matters and while disagreement lingers over the specific limits, there seems to be a strong consensus that physicians should not abandon their *primary* role as patient advocate.[2] Thus, the focus here is on the duties of the other stakeholders and how they can help to foster an environment where physicians can deliver quality care with the fewest possible impediments in the context of the new health care environment.

ORGANIZATIONAL RESPONSIBILITIES

Beginning on a broad scale, managed care organizations should be held to behavioral standards which are consistent with the objective of service to the community through the provision of quality health care, in return for a *reasonable* profit (or "surplus"). Such a purpose is consistent with an enlightened model of business and with the realities of medicine as it has predominantly been practiced by individual physicians. Moreover, these objectives are almost always expressed outright in the mission statements and promotional materials of corporations. No corporation offering a managed care plan expresses "profit maximization through cost-cutting initiatives within the sole parameters of law" as its stated purpose. Based upon these mission statements alone, the conclusion can be drawn that stakeholders, such as patients, physicians, and the surrounding community, should be important parts of the planning and decision process if these organizations are to act in a manner which is in accordance with their own expressed purposes.

With these broad objectives in mind, Rawlsian principles of fairness have clear implications in terms of balancing stakeholder interests and governing the specific behavior of managed care organizations. Consistent with the overall progression of medicine towards greater patient involvement in decision making, managed care organizations have duties to engage in the complete disclosure of plan contract terms and to end controversial practices such as "gag orders" which limit patient access to important information.[3]

Such restrictions are clearly immoral and should be proscribed as a matter of social policy. Fairness and respect for persons demand that patients have access to information such as non-covered treatment options and physician remuneration arrangements. Although fuller disclosure will not lead to a perfect market relationship of equal parties, the availability of such information will move the relationship closer to that ideal. It is also more consistent with the traditional medical doctrine of informed consent, since it will allow patients to make informed choices over whether or not to appeal a treatment denial or to pay for the procedure through other resources.

Disclosing remuneration information will also foster patient awareness of potential financial conflicts of interest on the part of their treating physicians. Patients have the right to know whether or not their physicians will gain by refraining from making a referral to a specialist or withholding an expensive procedure. A clear benefit of this type of disclosure is that physicians will be forced to exercise caution before acting in a manner which favors their own interests, because they will know that patients have access to such information. There is precedent for such disclosure in some traditional business settings, where the consumer must be provided with information about practices or products which have potentially adverse consequences.[4] Although disclosure is not required for every possible harm in typical commercial settings, most other businesses do not have human life so readily at stake. Thus, there is no inherent conflict in assigning these duties to managed care organizations.

When specific procedures are not covered by contract or are denied under the guise of "experimental" care, the principle of fairness demands that there are adequate mechanisms in place to appeal denied claims. Moreover, the label "investigative" or "experimental" must not be employed in a descriptive manner so overly broad that effective treatments are excluded. While having all such procedures articulated in advance would be preferable, there will always be conflict over the clinical value versus the cost of specific procedures, especially given rapidly changing technology. Consequently, the focus should be placed on the development of an adequate *process* to properly address these questions in a manner not biased toward the organizational goal of profit.[5] The exclusive use of independent reviewers for these types of decisions must be encouraged.

Managed care organizations have further moral responsibilities to continue to work with employers in order to develop quality and performance measurement tools which include information on specific quality measures as well as data on enrollee satisfaction, utilization, financial indicators, and access to care.[6] Clearly, the goal of assured quality is critical to the ability to reduce costs safely without jeopardizing patient health.[7] The development of accurate quality measurement methods has the potential of giving real meaning to the term "investigative" in determining the effectiveness of specific procedures. If made widely available, such data also gives patients much more power to make important distinctions among plans. Adequate measurements of quality are still in their infancy and will probably never reach a state where they can, or should, consistently supersede physician judgment.[8] However, the development of such measures is critical to a health care system that is attempting to curb spending while maintaining adequate degrees of quality and patient choice. Thus, managed care organizations have an obligation to continue their efforts in contributing to initiatives to improve these measures.

Paying physicians through capitation plans is another controversial practice in which ethical duties must be developed for organizations. Many observers believe these types of arrangements should be legally banned; they believe that when a doctor agrees to treat a load of patients in exchange for a fixed monthly sum, there are insurmountable temptations to skimp on care since the physician's financial well-being is directly on the line.

While these are understandable concerns, we must be clear that no method of payment, including salary, is completely free from the potential for a financial conflict of interest. While capitation arrangements change the specific nature of the tension, they do not introduce a new ethical problem to medicine. David Orentlicher notes that in most cases, these incentives may not unjustly limit care because of professional norms, the threat of malpractice, and the cost effectiveness of preventative treatments that curtail higher costs later.[9]

Furthermore, in light of the fact that there is a tremendous need to reduce wasteful spending, capitation may be the least invasive way to encourage the practice of cost-effective medicine while maintaining clinical freedom for physicians. In lieu of these arrangements, micro-management through various forms of utilization review for routine care must be heavily employed to control costs.[10] While it would be ideal if cost cutting could be accomplished through a process whereby physicians follow a comprehensive procedure manual and only prescribe care which is truly needed and effective, no such "cookbook" covering every possible ailment exists. Thus, either physicians or utilization reviewers must make judgment calls regarding treatments. These arrangements preserve practice autonomy by giving physicians the freedom to make these decisions in conjunction with patients. In addition, as Mariner points out, when some of the potential for financial loss is shifted to the physician, an MCO's financial interest is rarely in conflict with the patient's. Rather, it is the individual physician who then faces the potential conflict.[11] As a result, capitation arrangements may be the lesser of evils. Rather than the elimination of the practice altogether, the more appropriate discussion should focus on how the practice should be carried out so that physician ethical conflicts are minimized and patient interests are best served.

Although capitation leaves the direct conflict in the hands of individual physicians, several ethical obligations can be assigned to managed care organizations, since the institutional pressure resulting from the structure of the arrangements can serve to either enhance or reduce the degree of the tension confronting doctors. To begin with, the amount of the payment itself is of critical importance. Consistent with claims made by spokespersons for managed care organizations, these payments must be adequate to truly cover the cost of patient care. If these amounts are in fact sufficient, physicians should be protected in advocating for their patients within these limits. Following the lead of organizations (such as U.S. Health Care), catastrophic insurance should also be made available to physicians who treat sicker patient loads and exceed their pre-set capitation limits.[12] This would relieve physicians from the tension, which may arise at the end of the fiscal period, to severely skimp on patient care in order to avoid either a loss of income or removal from a provider panel.

In addition, many arrangements use bonuses and withhold "at risk" amounts until the end of a fiscal period. The amount of ancillary payment may make a difference with respect to the strength of potential conflicts of interest that may occur. In general, the larger the amount withheld, the greater the pressures will be to withhold needed care.[13] However, these ancillary payments are usually determined in conjunction with a "risk pool" which may further affect decision making.[14]

The greater the amount withheld and the more individualized the risk pool, the stronger the potential for conflicts will be. It is critical that the withheld amount is relatively low and the actual risk is spread across a group of physicians, so that unconscionable situations, in which the withholding of an expensive treatment directly results in more take-home pay, are clearly avoided. Finally, specific screens must be established to ensure that physicians are not skimping on quality or preventative care procedures in order to maximize their own income.

Managed care organizations also have moral obligations to refrain from the use of certain types of claims in their persuasive advertising and promotional materials used to attract new members. Moreover, they should participate in initiatives with surrounding public sector institutions to establish information disclosure standards that help enrollees differentiate plans on the basis of real quality distinctions. This information should be made widely available to the public through the use of uniform standards. The Fair Labeling and Packaging Act for food products could be used as a model to help consumers make sense of claims of better care.

Curbing certain types of persuasive claims and the use of uniform information is consistent with the variable "reasonable consumer" standard used to regulate advertising in traditional business settings. The typical potential enrollee for managed care can be more easily misled with respect to advertisements for health care than he or she might be for other consumer goods. Claims for "better quality care" are especially misleading, since there is broad disagreement over how this is best measured.[15] Self-imposed restrictions on advertising are by no means inconsistent with the "business" side of the organizations.[16] There are precedents for voluntary restrictions in other traditional commercial settings. For example, the software industry recently formed a group to address questionable marketing tactics by some members of its industry.[17] Wine makers have had an effective self-developed and enforced code for responsible advertising in place for a number of years.[18]

Finally, managed care organizations must also refrain from the temptation to increase profits by skimping on preventative care and engaging in "cherry picking," namely, insuring only the healthiest members of society. One possible public policy method to address these problems is "risk sharing" among insurers. Similar to "assigned risk pools" for automobile insurance in certain states, each managed care plan, depending on size, could be assigned an allotment of higher-risk patients. This will work simultaneously to protect patients and to ensure some amount of fairness among plans. In knowing that some patients with higher health costs will be assigned to them, managed care organizations will have direct incentives to engage in preventative care. However, these institutions are only one part of a larger social system. Thus, other stakeholders also have important responsibilities.

COMMUNITY/GOVERNMENTAL RESPONSIBILITIES

Following Adam Smith's conception of the need for equal players and the legitimacy of judicial enforcement in an efficient marketplace, there is a proper place for community intervention through governmental action to set the broad parameters for managed care organizations. Because medicine is an arena in which there are asymmetries of bargaining power, the community should act through the government to equalize the footing of the various stakeholders in places where the market clearly falls short.

First, as mentioned earlier, it is a community responsibility to provide health care for the indigent. Clearly, medicine is in that category of public goods such as food, safety, and education, which are necessary to sustain a reasonable quality of life. Thus, rather than clamoring against the greed of managed care organizations for not providing this good without recompense, the community has a duty to provide a "decent minimum" in terms of access to health care for citizens.[19] While there are clear disagreements over what qualifies as "decent" and over whether or not such care should be solely funded through public resources, these are merely secondary issues to the responsibility of acknowledging that such a duty exists.[20]

Through public agencies, the community also has a responsibility to work in conjunction with managed care organizations and employers on initiatives which establish quality measures and information disclosure standards so that enrollees can accurately make distinctions among plans. There is a great danger that employers and managed care organizations may share a primary agenda of cost-savings. Thus, the broader community must be involved in these initiatives to ensure that such standards are not unfairly biased in favor of these interests.

In addition to these responsibilities, the concept of fairness mandates the closure of regulatory loopholes such as the ERISA exemption and the provision of uniform regulatory standards. As noted in chapter 1, ERISA has permitted organizations that have committed serious wrongdoing to escape certain forms of liability by removing state-level legal remedies for patients. For example, in the case of *Corcoran v United Health Care*, a patient who lost her unborn fetus due to a faulty decision on the part of her employer's utilization review company discovered that she had almost no rights for redress. Because she was under an employer-sponsored health care plan, her case was the exclusive domain of ERISA, effectively removing her right to sue the plan under state tort laws. Clearly, organizations as organizations are not adequately being held responsible for their actions with the presence of such an escape mechanism. Furthermore, the ideal of a level playing field is violated when harmed patients are left without sufficient legal remedies even to approximate conditions under which they are able to punish unscrupulous actors. As the *Corcoran* court stated, serious mistakes could wind up being cost-free to the organizations that make them.[21] This is an unacceptable outcome even in a *laissez-faire* model of the marketplace.

An additional community responsibility is the establishment of minimum standards for covered treatments. Given rapid changes in technology, these standards should be frequently updated. As a society, we have decided that there are minimal levels of safety standards for most products and services. The range of risk for which a consumer is free to contract is clearly limited. Similar requirements should be established for managed care plans, particularly in light of the fact that patients are at a much greater disadvantage because it is much more difficult to predict adequately their own needs for health care than for other goods. In chapter 7, a managed care executive was quoted as stating that because of financial disadvantages, his organization could not pay for cutting-edge cancer research if his competitors did not. Insisting upon a level playing field for all managed care organizations, this executive stated further that "if you want to do it through a tax, that's fine."[22] While his statement focused on research funding, coverage for expensive standard and experimental procedures and emergency care presents similar dilemmas. Thus, the community should establish and enforce minimum acceptable levels of care and covered procedures. This is the only way of breaking insular standoffs among managed care organizations that could result in significant harm to patients.

Through legislative measures, the community should also establish qualifications for, and clarify the role of, utilization reviewers. Many decisions over experimental procedures go beyond the scope of whether or not a therapy is covered by the plan, and into the more ambiguous territory of effectiveness versus cost. Since it is currently illegal for non-physicians to practice medicine, it is clear that doctors must play a significant role in the review process. Legislatures must examine this process and establish clearer standards with respect to the personnel who are engaged in making these decisions.

Moreover, the true independence of review organizations should be established and maintained. The primary service obligations of utilization review companies ought to be clarified. The independence of the utilization review firm hired by the managed care organization must be established by law. Otherwise, there is a built-in conflict of interest; the review agency may err in favor of the managed care organization to avoid being discharged for granting too many approvals. Standards for the relationship between utilization review organizations and the managed care organizations which contract with them should be established by the broader society.[23] There is some precedent in business settings for such an independent role. For example, in conducting audits of financial statements, public accountants are in fact held to the standard of serving "the public" rather than the organizations that remunerate them for their services.

The community must also address the issue of high turnover rates due to changes in either employment status or employer. In addition to the problems of broken continuity with physicians and the lack of consistent medical records, high turnover increases the potential for some managed care organizations to "cherry pick" and to skimp on preventative care.[24] Although the available evi-

dence suggests that these are not common practices, the temptation is undeniably present. With current turnover rates, it would
be easy to protect financial resources by insuring only healthy
members of the population and to refrain from spending on preventative care, because there is a good chance that long-term
benefits will accrue to another plan.

The community should also make strident efforts to avoid
blaming managed care organizations for the developing cost-
consciousness in medicine. Financial considerations would be a
part of the new health care environment in the absence of managed care. Furthermore, before misguided policies are enacted by
policymakers and voters, it is critical that responsibility for decisions such as denials of care is properly assigned. As mentioned
earlier, managed care organizations are often incorrectly blamed
for decisions that are actually made by hospitals, practice groups,
or individual physicians. Thus, while voters may be angry at the
changing nature of medical delivery, legal proposals and ballot initiatives will not solve their concerns if the wrong entities are targeted.

Finally, while there is a legitimate role for community intervention, there is also a responsibility to refrain from the over-exten-
sion of such authority. The market mechanism should be allowed
to function freely where it will legitimately lead to improvements in health care. Several plans have responded to demands
for broader choices and are beginning to offer enrollees the ability of visiting out-of-network physicians and/or the option of self-
referral to see specialists in exchange for higher out-of-pocket
fees. While the fees may still be too high for some patients, there
is potential that competition will force these rates downward as
other plans lower them in order to attract patients. Thus, market
forces should be allowed to work where they can.

EMPLOYER RESPONSIBILITIES

As the primary purchasers of care, employers play a significant
part in the current health care equation. Rather than exclusively
focusing on seeking the least expensive plan, they have a moral responsibility to consider the health of their employees. They should

follow the example of the growing number of corporations that are participating in quality improvement and accreditation initiatives.[25] This participation is reflective of an enlightened model of employee relations which has been embraced by many corporations. For example, many organizations had family-leave policies in place long before the federal act mandated such practices.[26] Moreover, numerous companies are moving toward other, flexible, family-friendly employment practices.[27] In fact, the argument can be made that these types of practices are actually "good business" because they boost morale and allow a company to save on the turnover costs associated with hiring new employees. Similarly, the extension of such policies to consider employee health needs would not bring a new dimension into business, especially since time taken off from work because of illness is a costly expense.

Employers should also educate their employees about the health care choices made during enrollment periods. Current contractual language is much too complex to be understood by the average lay person. Thus, employers should assist in this process, and help their employees make appropriate distinctions between plan options.

PATIENT RESPONSIBILITIES

The new medical environment mandates that patients, as the end-recipients of care, bear greater moral responsibilities than they have in the past. Patients must take more responsibility for their own health. In addition to the practice of good health-related habits, they should take advantage of the preventative care offered by managed care organizations so that illnesses are detected and treated as early as possible. Patients who choose not to take advantage of such services, or who ignore their physician's advice about lifestyle behaviors, are acting at the direct expense of themselves and others.

Patients must learn as much as they can about their managed care arrangements so that they can function as knowledgeable patients. This will result in the improvement of their abilities to advocate for themselves in the new health care environment. Lastly, they must change their paradigms and realize that health care is not a "free" benefit. Waste on their part necessarily means that less will be left for others. The principle of fairness to others mandates that we must all do our share to be judicious in the utilization of medical resources. Thus, patients must refrain from frivolous use, and exercise responsibility in appealing what they take to be unjust economic constraints on their care.[28]

CONCLUSION

The ethical challenges in the new health care environment are undoubtedly great. Patients and physicians are accustomed to a situation where all claims for medical procedures are honored and the ensuing expenses are covered by third-party payers. Managed care organizations are engaged in the difficult task of reducing health care spending while maintaining high levels of quality.

These organizations are attempting to serve in dual roles as businesses and as entities engaged in the delivery of medicine. While they have stabilized aggregate-level medical costs, some of their current practices indicate that the health of individual patients may be harmed in the process. Without a moral framework that accounts for both roles, several dangers exist. First, these types of practices may continue unabated, and some profits will be made at the direct expense of the quality of patient care offered. Second, there is a distinct possibility that as a reaction to these practices, legislation will be passed that overly restricts these organizations, and thereby prevents them from contributing to the goals of improved patient care and lower aggregate costs.

An adequate moral grounding, however, cannot be found in the traditional understanding either of medical or of business ethics, because neither offers behavioral guidelines that account for both of these organizational roles. The traditional patient-centered ethic is unrealistic and irresponsible within the climate of resource limits, and a laissez-faire model of business cannot properly protect the interests of patients, physicians, and other important constituents.

In contrast, an enlightened stakeholder approach offers much promise as an ethical framework to govern the behavior of managed care organizations as businesses engaged in the delivery of medicine. Within such an approach, these organizations can be expected to honor moral duties going well beyond the maximization of shareholder wealth. In addition, ethical obligations can be further assigned to other important stakeholders because they share a reciprocal relationship with these organizations and they play critical roles in the new health care environment.

Working together, managed care organizations along with other stakeholders can endeavor to ensure that health care delivery is shaped in a manner that honors the best interests of society, rather than irresponsible claims for individual treatment or short-term financial goals of physicians and organizations. If the moral obligations of each of these parties are consistently carried out, managed care offers society its best hope of achieving a more just medical delivery system. Although ethical conflicts will still undoubtedly arise, these organizations can simultaneously maintain a high level of quality for individual patients, while improving broader access to care by curbing costs. In so doing, the normative principles of justice articulated by John Rawls will be best balanced. The greatest amount of liberty possible will be retained by both patients and physicians, while health care will be made more readily available for the millions of members of society who currently have no access to coverage at all.

Notes

INTRODUCTION

1. David R. Olmos, "Cutting Health Costs or Corners?" *Los Angeles Times*, 5 May 1995, A1; and Erik Larson, "The Soul of an HMO," *Time*, 22 January 1996, 45–52.

2. See Wendy K. Mariner, "Business vs. Medical Ethics: Conflicting Standards for Managed Care," *Journal of Law, Medicine & Ethics* 23 (1995): 236–246.

3. Bettijane Levine, "He Might Have the Cure for Medicine's Ills" (interview with Lonnie Bristow), *Los Angeles Times*, 18 July 1995, E1.

4. See Alain C. Enthoven and Sara J. Singer, "2010 Will Be Too Late to Reform," *Los Angeles Times*, 12 March 1997, B3. See also Enthoven and Richard Kronick, "Universal Health Insurance through Incentives Reform," *Journal of the American Medical Association* 265, no. 19 (15 May 1991): 2532.

5. See Paul M. Ellwood, Jr., and George D. Lundberg, "Managed Care: A Work in Progress," *Journal of the American Medical Association* 276, no. 13 (2 October 1996): 1083–1086; Enthoven and Kronick, "Universal Health Insurance"; and Michael McGarvey, "The Case for Managed Care," *Trends in Health Care, Law, & Ethics* 10, no. 1/2 (Winter/Spring 1995): 45–46.

6. See Edmund D. Pellegrino, "Allocation of Resources at the Bedside: The Intersections of Economics, Law, and Ethics," *Kennedy Institute of Ethics Journal* 4, no. 4 (1994): 312. For a similar perspective, see Ruth Macklin, *Enemies of Patients* (New York: Oxford University Press, 1993), 147–165.

7. The perspective that only non-profits should be engaged in the delivery of care is one which is growing in popularity. See Kate T. Christensen, "Ethically Important Distinctions among Managed Care Organizations," *Journal of Law, Medicine & Ethics* 23 (1995): 223–239; and Pellegrino, "Interests, Obligations, and Justice: Some Notes toward

an Ethic of Managed Care," *Journal of Clinical Ethics* 6, no. 4 (Winter 1995): 316.

8. See Nancy Jecker, "Managed Competition and Managed Care: What Are the Ethical Issues?" *Clinics in Geriatric Medicine* 10, no. 3 (August 1994): 527–540; and Ruth Macklin, "The Ethics of Managed Care," *Trends in Health Care, Law & Ethics* 10, no. 1/2 (Winter/Spring 1995): 63–66.

9. See Arnold Relman and Uwe Reinhardt, "An Exchange on For-Profit Health Care," in Institute of Medicine, *For-Profit Enterprise in Health Care* (Washington, D.C.: National Academy Press, 1986), 209–223. In this discussion, Reinhardt unsuccessfully challenges Relman to give a positive description of what he believes would be a more ethical program for reform.

10. See *Wickline v State of California*, 239 Cal. Rptr. 810 (Ct. App. 1986).

11. Susan Wolf, "Towards a Theory of Process," *Law, Medicine, & Health Care* 20, no. 4 (Winter 1992): 278–290.

12. Susan Wolf, "Health Care Reform and the Future of Physician Ethics," *Hastings Center Report* 24, no. 2 (1994): 28–41; also see Ezekial J. Emanual, "Medical Ethics in the Era of Managed Care: The Need for Institutional Structures instead of Principles for Individual Cases," *Journal of Clinical Ethics* 6, no. 4 (1995): 335–338.

13. See Phillip M. Nudelman and Linda M. Andrews, "The 'Value Added' of Not-for-Profit Health Plans," *New England Journal of Medicine* 334, no. 16 (18 April 1996): 1057–1059; Christensen, "Ethically Important Distinctions among Managed Care Organizations," 223; and Carolyn M. Clancy and Howard Brody, "Managed Care: Jekyll or Hyde?" *Journal of the American Medical Association* 273, no. 4 (25 January 1995): 338–339.

14. Mariner, 238.

15. Uwe E. Reinhardt, "Managed Competition in Health Care Reform: Just Another American Dream, or the Perfect Solution?" *The Journal of Law, Medicine & Ethics* 22, no. 2 (Summer 1994): 109.

16. John Rawls, *A Theory of Justice* (Cambridge, Mass.: Harvard University Press, 1971).

17. Michael Sandel and Susan Okin are among the many notable critics of Rawls's foundational assumptions.

18. John Rawls, *Political Liberalism* (New York: Columbia University Press, 1993).

1. A detailed discussion of such profit-seeking behavior is given in Marc A. Rodwin, *Medicine, Money, and Morals* (New York: Oxford University Press, 1993).

2. Adapted from John K. Inglehart, "The American Health Care System: Managed Care," *New England Journal of Medicine* 327, no. 10 (3 September 1992): 742.

3. Nancy Jecker, "Managed Competition and Managed Care: What Are the Ethical Issues?" *Clinics in Geriatric Medicine* 10, no. 3 (August 1994): 529.

4. Inglehart, "The American Health Care System," 744.

5. Ibid.

6. Thomas J. Maxwell, "Health Reform/Managed Care: A View from a Doctor's Office," *Delaware Lawyer* (Spring 1995): 34.

7. Alain C. Enthoven and Richard Kronick, "Universal Health Insurance through Incentives Reform," *Journal of the American Medical Association* 265, no. 19 (15 May 1991): 2532.

8. Robert A. Rosenblatt, "Republicans Devise Plan to Cap Open-Ended Medicare Outlays," *Los Angeles Times*, 19 July 1995, A5.

9. John K. Inglehart, "The Struggle between Managed Care and Fee-for-Service Medicine," *New England Journal of Medicine* 331, no. 1 (7 July 1994): 65.

10. Michael A. Hiltzik and David Olmos, "A Mixed Diagnosis for HMO's," *Los Angeles Times*, 7 August 1995, A1.

11. Carolyn Long Engelhard and James F. Childress, "Caveat Emptor: The Cost of Managed Care," *Trends in Health Care, Law, & Ethics* 10, no. 1/2 (Winter/Spring 1995): 14.

12. Suzanne Gordon and Ellen D. Baer, "Keeping Quiet on the Tough Choices," *Los Angeles Times*, 24 January 1995, B7.

13. This is the amount withheld regardless of the initial payment method: salary, fee-for-service, or capitation. However, the practice of withholding is more customary in fee-for-service and capitation arrangements. For a more comprehensive discussion of these practices, see Alan Hillman, "Financial Incentives for Physicians in HMO's," *New England Journal of Medicine* 317, no. 27 (1987): 1743–1749.

14. David R. Olmos, "Cutting Health Costs or Corners?" *Los Angeles Times,* 5 May 1995, A1.

15. Ibid., A22.

16. Paul Elias, "Trial No Longer a Managed Care Test," *Los Angeles Times,* 10 November 1995, A3.

17. Ibid.

18. Suzanne Gordon, "Hippocratic or Hypocratic Oath?" *Los Angeles Times,* 21 January 1996, M5.

19. David R. Olmos and Shari Roan, "HMO Gag Clauses on Doctors Spur Protest," *Los Angeles Times,* 14 April 1996, A1.

20. Marc A. Rodwin, "Dealing with Conflicts of Interest in Managed Care," *New England Journal of Medicine* 332, no. 9 (2 March 1995): 605.

21. It is interesting to note that Kaiser is chartered as a non-profit corporation. As such, the organization has no obligations to distribute profits to third parties such as shareholders. Yet, in this case and in several others, the organization found itself under fire for cost-cutting and alleged "corporate greed." Such controversies have contributed to concerns that with the influx of for-profit corporations into medical care, non-profits are being forced to behave like their profit-seeking counterparts in order to compete and survive, further eroding the traditional focus on patient well-being.

22. Charles E. Schmidt, Jr., "Managed Care Faces Stinging Backlash," *Best's Review* (November 1995): 22.

23. Robert Rosenblatt, "Federal Mandates in Health Insurance Alarm Providers," *Los Angeles Times,* 3 October 1996, D1.

24. Erik Larson, "The Soul of an HMO," *Time,* 22 January 1996, 44–52.

25. Michael Hiltzik, "HMO Slapped with $1-Million Judgment in Cancer Case," *Los Angeles Times,* 18 October 1996, D1.

26. Ibid.

27. Edmund D. Pellegrino, "Allocation of Resources at the Bedside: The Intersections of Economics, Law, and Ethics," *Kennedy Institute of Ethics Journal* 4, no. 4 (1994): 312. For a similar perspective, see Ruth Macklin, *Enemies of Patients* (New York: Oxford University Press, 1993), 147–165.

28. Arnold S. Relman, "Medical Practice under the Clinton Reforms: Avoiding Domination by Big Business," *New England Journal of Medicine* 329, no. 21 (18 November 1993): 1574–1576.

29. M. Stanton Evans et al., "The Trouble with HMO's," *Consumers' Research*, July 1995, 12.

30. Paul T. Menzel, "Economic Competition in Health Care: A Moral Assessment," *Journal of Medicine and Philosophy* 12 (1987): 63–84.

31. Allan S. Brett, "The Case against Persuasive Advertising by Health Maintenance Organizations," *New England Journal of Medicine* 326, no. 20 (14 May 1992): 1353–1356.

32. "Managed Care," Segment from NBC Evening News Broadcast, 11 April 1996.

33. Dan W. Brock and Allen E. Buchanan, "The Profit Motive in Medicine," *Journal of Medicine and Philosophy* 12 (1987): 1–35. Although Brock and Buchanan argue in support of for-profit enterprises in medicine, they give a detailed discussion of the moral issues raised by the elimination of cost-shifting/cross-subsidization practices.

34. David R. Olmos, "HMO Cites $20 Million in Failed-Merger Costs," *Los Angeles Times*, 13 February 1996, D3.

35. Wendy K. Mariner, "Business vs. Medical Ethics: Conflicting Standards for Managed Care," *Journal of Law, Medicine & Ethics* 23 (1995): 243.

36. Mitchell T. Rabkin, "Targeting and Coordinating the Incentives," *New England Journal of Medicine* 309, no. 16 (20 October 1983): 982–984.

37. E. Haavi Morreim, "Moral Justice and Legal Justice in Managed Care: The Ascent of Contributive Justice," *Journal of Law, Medicine & Ethics* 23 (1995): 247–265.

38. David R. Olmos, "Cutting Health Costs or Corners?" *Los Angeles Times*, 5 May 1995, A22.

39. Malik Hasan, "Let's End the Non-Profit Charade," *New England Journal of Medicine* 334, no. 16 (18 April 1996): 1055–1057.

40. See Lloyd M. Krieger, "How Managed Care Will Allow Market Forces to Solve the Problems," *New York Times*, 13 August 1995, F12(L); and J. D. Kleinke, "Triumph of the Market," *Barron's*, 24 October 1994, 59.

41. Quoted in Julie Kosterlitz, "Unmanaged Care?" *National Journal* (10 December 1994): 2904.

42. Schmidt, 84.

43. Jerome P. Kassirer, "Managed Care and the Morality of the Marketplace," *New England Journal of Medicine* 333, no. 1 (6 July 1995): 50.

44. David C. Thomasma, "The Ethics of Managed Care and Cost Con-

trol," *Trends in Health Care, Law & Ethics* 10, no. 1/2 (Winter/Spring 1995): 33.

45. Inglehart, "The Struggle between Managed Care and Fee-for-Service Practice," 66.

46. Leigh Page, "Market Spawns Doctor-Patient Alliances," *American Medical News* 38, no. 42 (13 November 1995): 3.

47. George Anders and Laura Johannes, "Doctors Are Losing a Lobbying Battle to HMO's," *Wall Street Journal*, 15 May 1995, B1. Also see Page, 3.

48. David R. Olmos, "Law Will Boost Terminal Patient's Rights," *Los Angeles Times*, 28 September 1996, A22.

49. See Page, 3.

50. For example, two initiatives appeared on the ballot for the November 1996 elections in California, the state in which managed care has made its greatest inroads. While neither passed, the initiatives would have limited some of the most controversial practices of the industry, such as financial incentives given to doctors or nurses to deny or delay care and the previously mentioned "gag orders" allegedly placed upon physicians. Prior to the vote, opponents of the initiatives argued that such measures would drive up taxes and the cost of health care without necessarily improving quality. As a result, they argued, some patients would be hurt since smaller employers would be forced to drop health care coverage altogether. See David R. Olmos, "2 Plans to Regulate HMO's Move toward Ballot," *Los Angeles Times*, 23 April 1996, A21.

51. While case law is not as powerful as legislative reforms, because courts of various levels and jurisdictions may reach conflicting opinions, it does provide another source of legal guidance for acceptable managed care practices.

52. Kathleen Sutherland Archuleta, "Integration of Health Care Delivery Systems: Potential Tort Liability," *Colorado Lawyer* 23, no. 8 (August 1994): 1808, note 3, citing the case of *Boyd v Albert Einstein Medical Center*, 547 A.2d 1229 (Pa. Super. 1988).

53. John G. Salmon, "Litigating Claims against Managed Health Care Organizations," *Trial* (February 1995): 81–82. Also see Archuleta, 1809–1810, for a detailed discussion of the *Wickline* and *Wilson* cases.

54. *Fox v Health Net*, Civ No. 219692 (Cal. Riverside County Superior Ct.,

December 28, 1993). See Salmon, 84, for a detailed discussion of this case.

55. In *Pilot Life v Dedeaux*, a court ruled that plaintiffs hoping to sue an MCO for a denial of benefit, which may even result in wrongful death, have no recourse under state measures and thus, they can recover only the original cost of the denied procedure. *Pilot Life Ins. Co. v Dedeaux*, 481 U.S. 41 (1987).

56. *Corcoran v United Health Care, Inc.*, 965 F.2d 1321 (5th Cir. 1992). See Kosterlitz for a detailed discussion of this case. Most recently, in a case which was decided in May 1995, the U.S. Supreme Court denied a suit in state court over allegations that Kaiser Foundation Health Plan had contributed to a patient's death by denying him an experimental treatment for cancer; see Michael Hiltzik, "Supreme Court Won't Allow Suit in Death Case," *Los Angeles Times*, 16 May 1995, D1.

57. See *Hand v Tavara*, No. 04-92-00618CV (4th Cir. September 22, 1993), cited in Alice Gosfield, "The Legal Subtext of the Managed Care Environment," *Journal of Law, Medicine & Ethics* 23 (1995): 231.

58. The seminal cases are *Wickline v State of California* (239 Cal. Rptr. 810 Ct. App. 1986) and *Wilson v Blue Cross of Southern California* (271 Cal. Rptr. 876 Ct. App. 1990), rehearing denied, October 11, 1990.

59. *Bush v Dake*, No. 86-25767 (Mich. Cir Ct. April 27, 1989). See Gosfield, 231.

60. *Hand v Tavara*, No. 04-92-00618CV (4th Cir. September 22, 1993).

61. *Fox v Health Net*, Civ. No. 219692 (Cal., Riverside County Super. Ct., December 28, 1993.)

62. Salmon, 84.

63. Schmidt, 22.

64. See Barry J. Furrow, "Managed Care and the Evolution of Quality," *Trends in Health Care, Law & Ethics* 10, no. 1/2 (Winter/Spring 1995): 38.

65. See also Morreim, "Moral Justice and Legal Justice in Managed Care." Although the author is against such a change, a detailed discussion of this issue is provided by Edward B. Hirshfield, "Should Ethical and Legal Standards for Physicians Be Changed to Accommodate New Models of Health Care?" *University of Pennsylvania Law Review* 140 (1992): 1809–1846.

66. *Harrell v Total Care, Inc.*, 781. S.W. 2d 58, 61 (Mo. 1989), quoted in Furrow, 38.

Two   REFRAMING THE DEBATE:
      PERSPECTIVES CRITICAL OF MANAGED CARE

1. See Nancy Jecker, "Managed Competition and Managed Care: What Are the Ethical Issues?" *Clinics in Geriatric Medicine* 10, no. 3 (August 1994): 527–540; and Ruth Macklin, "The Ethics of Managed Care," *Trends in Health Care, Law & Ethics* 10, no. 1/2 (Winter/Spring 1995): 63–66.

2. It is important to note that I have not drawn the horizontal axis as a simple choice between fee-for-service and managed care. Contrary to how the debate is represented in much of the current literature, fee-for-service arrangements are present (typically on a discounted scale) in some types of managed care plans.

3. Ezekial J. Emanuel and Nancy Neveloff Dubler, "Preserving the Physician-Patient Relationship in an Era of Managed Care," *Journal of the American Medical Association* 273, no. 4 (25 January 1995): 326–329.

4. See William V. Healey, "The Ethics of Managed Care," *Business Ethics* (November/December 1994): 8–9.

5. See John K. Inglehart, "The Struggle between Managed Care and Fee-for-Service Medicine," *New England Journal of Medicine* 331, no. 1 (7 July 1994): 63–67.

6. Edmund D. Pellegrino, "Words Can Hurt You: Some Reflections on the Metaphors of Managed Care," First Annual Nicholas Pisano Lecture, *Journal of the American Board of Family Practice* 7, no. 6 (November–December 1994): 508. It is important to note that Pellegrino has given some support for non-profit managed care organizations in his more recent work on the subject. However, it appears that this represents an acknowledgment of the realities of the growth of these plans rather than his ideal model for health care delivery. See Pellegrino, "Interests, Obligations, and Justice: Some Notes toward an Ethic of Managed Care," *Journal of Clinical Ethics* 6, no. 4 (Winter 1995): 316. Also see Macklin, "The Ethics of Managed Care," 63–66.

7. Healey, 8–9.

8. John W. Merline, "Making Money by Denying Care," *Consumers' Research*, September 1994, 10–15.

9. For example, see Edmund Pellegrino, "Ethics," *Journal of the American Medical Association* 271, no. 21 (1 June 1994): 1668–1670.

10. See Joseph Fins, "The Hidden Costs of Market-Based Health Care Reform," *Hastings Center Report* (May–June 1992): 6.

11. Sam J. Sugar, Letter to the Editor, *New England Journal of Medicine* 333, no. 18 (2 November 1995): 1220.

12. See Pellegrino, "Words Can Hurt You: Some Reflections on the Metaphors of Managed Care," 505–510.

13. Jerome P. Kassirer, "Managed Care and the Morality of the Marketplace," *New England Journal of Medicine* 333, no. 1 (6 July 1995): 51.

14. Theodore R. Marmor and Jerry L. Mashaw, "Madison Ave. Meets Marcus Welby," *Los Angeles Times*, 19 February 1995, M5.

15. Joseph Sullivan, "Officials Scrutinizing Doctor Bonuses in Managed Care Plans," *New York Times*, 21 September 1995, B6(L).

16. See Paul T. Menzel, "Economic Competition in Health Care: A Moral Assessment," *Journal of Medicine and Philosophy* 12 (1987): 63–84; and Robert Pear, "H.M.O.'s Refusing Emergency Claims, Hospitals Assert," *New York Times*, 9 July 1995, A1.

17. Carolyn Long Engelhard and James F. Childress, "Caveat Emptor: The Cost of Managed Care," *Trends in Health Care, Law & Ethics* 10, no. 1/2 (Winter/Spring 1995): 13.

18. Emanuel and Dubler, "Preserving the Physician-Patient Relationship in an Era of Managed Care," 326.

19. Ezekial J. Emanuel and Allan S. Brett, "Managed Competition and the Patient-Physician Relationship," *New England Journal of Medicine* 329, no. 12 (16 September 1993): 880.

20. Emanuel and Dubler, 326. Also see Jim Schachter, "Insured People Satisfied with Medical Care," *Los Angeles Times*, 28 August 1995, A1.

21. Although Relman supports the development of community-based, physician-owned managed care organizations, he has expressed this common criticism. See Arnold S. Relman, "Medical Practice under the Clinton Reforms: Avoiding Domination by Big Business," *Journal of the American Medical Association* 329, no. 21 (18 November 1993): 1574. Also see Alice Gosfield, "The Legal Subtext of the Managed Care Environment: A Practitioner's Perspective," *Journal of Law, Medicine & Ethics* 23 (1995): 235. Although Gosfield does not state that she supports a return to fee-for-service medicine, she argues that patient satisfaction surveys are inadequate measures of quality.

22. Bruce Vladeck, "Medicare Has No Use for Managed Care," *New York Times*, 14 June 1995, A24(L).

23. Council on Ethical and Judicial Affairs, American Medical Association, "Ethical Issues in Managed Care," *Journal of the American Medical Association* 273, no. 4 (25 January 1995): 330–335.

24. Inglehart, "The Struggle between Managed Care and Fee-for-Service Medicine," 66.

25. Ibid., 64.

26. Sherman B. Child, "Managed Care," Letter to the Editor, *New England Journal of Medicine* 333, no. 18 (2 November 1995): 1219.

27. J. Patrick Rooney, "Medisave in Practice: An Insurer's Example," *Consumers' Research*, March 1992, 12–13.

28. John C. Goodman, "A Plan to Empower Patients," *Wall Street Journal*, 2 May 1995, A24, col. 3.

29. David E. Kim, Letter to the Editor, *New England Journal of Medicine* 333, no. 18 (2 November 1995): 1220.

30. Murray Weidenbaum, "Can the Free Market Cure America's Health Care Disease?" *Business and Society Review* 93 (Spring 1995): 26–32.

31. See Weidenbaum, 27, and John C. Goodman and Gerald L. Musgrave, "How to Solve the Health Care Crisis," *Consumers' Research*, March 1992, 11.

32. W. G. Manning et al., "Health Insurance and the Demand for Health Care," *American Economic Review* (June 1987): 251–277, cited in Kenneth E. Thorpe, "Medical Savings Accounts: Design and Policy Issues," *Health Affairs* 14, no. 3 (1995): 254–259.

33. Weidenbaum, 26–32.

34. Child, 1219.

35. Goodman, "A Plan to Empower Patients," A24, col. 3.

36. Goodman and Musgrave, "How to Solve the Health Care Crisis," 10–14, 35.

37. Ibid., 12.

38. Ibid., 11.

39. These figures are based upon claims in Chicago, one of the nation's highest claim areas. In other areas, only about 9 percent of claims exceed $2,000, quoted in Michael Tanner, "Returning Medicine to

the Marketplace," in *Market Liberalism*, ed. David Boaz and Edward Crane (Washington, D.C.: Cato Institute, 1993), 185–186.

40. Rooney uses the example of a plan with a $3,000 deductible that can be purchased for $1,500. See Rooney, 12–13.

41. Ibid., 13.

42. Tanner, 186.

43. Rooney, 13, and Tanner, 186.

44. Lonnie R. Bristow, "Let's Not Rule Out Managed Care Accounts," Letter to the Editor, *New York Times*, 9 October 1995, A10(N).

45. Sheryl Stolberg, "Dole's Push for Health Savings Accounts Defeated," *Los Angeles Times*, 19 April 1996, A1.

46. For a detailed explanation of these concerns, see David Orentlicher, "Managed Care and the Threat to the Patient-Physician Relationship," *Trends in Health Care, Law & Ethics* 10, no. 1/2 (Winter/Spring 1995): 19–24.

47. For a good overview of these arguments, see Arthur L. Caplan, "Can Money and Morality Mix in Medicine?" *Academic Emergency Medicine* 1, no. 1 (January/February 1994): 75; and Richard D. Lamm, "Managed Care Heresies," *Trends in Health Care, Law & Ethics* 10, no. 1/2 (Winter/Spring 1995): 15–18, 72.

48. See David C. Thomasma, "The Ethics of Managed Care and Cost Control," *Trends in Health Care, Law & Ethics* 10, no. 1/2 (Winter/Spring 1995): 33–36, 44.

49. Daniel Callahan, *Setting Limits: Medical Goals in an Aging Society* (New York: Simon & Schuster, 1987).

50. See David Mechanic, "Professional Judgment and the Rationing of Medical Care," *University of Pennsylvania Law Review* 140 (1992): 1740. Mechanic cites Henry J. Aaron and William B. Schwartz, *The Painful Prescription: Rationing Hospital Care* (Washington, D.C.: Brookings Institution, 1984).

51. See Robert Blank, "The Regulatory Model: Rationing Health Care," *University of Pennsylvania Law Review* (1992): 1573, cited in Mechanic, 1722. Also see Caplan, 76.

52. See for example, Daniel Callahan, "Ethics and Priority Setting in Oregon," *Health Affairs* 10, no. 2 (Summer 1991).

53. For a further description, see David C. Hadorn, "The Oregon Prior-

ity-Setting Exercise: Quality of Life and Public Policy," *Hastings Center Report* 21, no. 3 (May–June 1991).

54. See E. Haavi Morreim, "Cost Containment: Challenging Fidelity and Justice," *Hastings Center Report* (December 1988): 22; Mechanic, 1720; and Caplan, 79–80. While Caplan states that he rejects rationing based upon his belief that we are not under conditions that justify its practice, he does support the development of "cookbooks" to save on expenditures.

55. See Robert M. Veatch, "DRG's and the Ethical Allocation of Resources," *Hastings Center Report* 32 (1986): 37–39, cited in Orentlicher, "Managed Care," 20. See also Caplan, 73–81. Although Caplan is morally unsupportive of explicit rationing at this point, he points out the bind that doctors are placed under in implicit rationing schemes such as gatekeeper arrangements. Caplan states that malpractice reform and reimbursement according to outcomes as established by "cookbooks" are a more ethical way to contain costs at the present time.

56. Thomasma, 33.

57. Lamm, 17.

58. Caplan, 77.

59. Thomasma, 61.

Three REFRAMING THE DEBATE: PERSPECTIVES IN SUPPORT OF MANAGED CARE

1. E. Haavi Morreim, "Moral Justice and Legal Justice in Managed Care: The Ascent of Contributive Justice," *Journal of Law, Medicine & Ethics* 23 (1995): 247–265.

2. See David Mechanic, "Professional Judgment and the Rationing of Medical Care," *University of Pennsylvania Law Review* 140, no. 1637 (1992), 1713–1754, and David Orentlicher, "Managed Care and the Threat to the Patient-Physician Relationship," *Trends in Health Care, Law & Ethics* 10, no. 1/2 (Winter/Spring 1995): 19–24.

3. Jeff C. Goldsmith et al., "Managed Care Comes of Age," *Healthcare Forum Journal* (September/October 1995): 16.

4. See Michael McGarvey, "The Case for Managed Care," *Trends in Health Care, Law & Ethics* 10, no. 1/2 (Winter/Spring 1995): 45–46, 52; and

Alain C. Enthoven and Richard Kronick, "Better Medicine at Lower Cost," *New York Times*, 12 June 1994, HR 6 (L).

5. Orentlicher, "Managed Care," 19–24.

6. Enthoven and Kronick, "Better Medicine at Lower Cost," HR 6 (L). Also see various writings by Paul Ellwood.

7. John LaPuma, Letter to the Editor, *Journal of the American Medical Association* 274, no. 8 (23/30 August 1995): 610.

8. See John T. Kelly and Shirley E. Kellie, "Appropriateness of Medical Care: Findings, Strategies," *Archives of Pathology & Laboratory Medicine* 114 (1990): 1119–1120, cited in Edward B. Hirshfield, "Should Ethical and Legal Standards for Physicians Be Changed to Accommodate New Models for Rationing Health Care?" *University of Pennsylvania Law Review* 140 (1992): 1821. See also Alain C. Enthoven and Richard Kronick, "Universal Health Insurance through Incentives Reform," *Journal of the American Medical Association* 265, no. 19 (15 May 1991): 2532–2536.

9. See Michael S. Broder, "In Health Care, We Cannot Have It All," *Los Angeles Times*, 27 December 1995, B9.

10. See Ezekial J. Emanuel and Nancy Neveloff Dubler, "Preserving the Physician-Patient Relationship in an Era of Managed Care," *Journal of the American Medical Association* 273, no. 4 (25 January 1995): 323–329; and E. Haavi Morreim, "Cost Containment: Challenging Fidelity and Justice," *Hastings Center Report* (December 1988): 20.

11. Mitchell Rabkin, "Control of Health Care Costs: Targeting and Co-ordinating the Incentives," *New England Journal of Medicine* 309, no. 16 (20 October 1993): 982–984.

12. Morreim, "Cost Containment: Challenging Fidelity and Justice," 20–25.

13. Thomas J. Maxwell, "Health Reform/Managed Care: A View from a Doctor's Office," *Delaware Lawyer* (Spring 1995): 36.

14. See McGarvey, 45; and Jecker, "Managed Competition and Managed Care: What Are the Ethical Issues?" *Clinics in Geriatric Medicine* 10, no. 3 (August 1994): 535.

15. Alain C. Enthoven, "In Defense of Managed Care," Letter to the Editor, *Wall Street Journal*, 17 February 1994, A17(E).

16. See Marc D. Hiller and James B. Lewis, "Managed Health Care Benefit Plans: What Are the Ethical Issues?" *Trends in Health Care, Law & Ethics*

10, no. 1/2 (Winter/Spring 1995): 109–112, 118; and McGarvey, 45–46, 53.

17. Group Health Association, *HMO Performance Reports* (Washington, D.C.: December 1994), cited in McGarvey, 46.

18. Arnold Relman and Uwe Reinhardt, "An Exchange on For-Profit Health Care," Institute of Medicine, *For-Profit Enterprise in Health Care* (Washington, D.C.: National Academy Press, 1986), 209–223.

19. McGarvey, 45–46, 53.

20. Dan W. Brock and Allen E. Buchanan, "The Profit Motive in Medicine," *Journal of Medicine and Philosophy* 12 (1987): 19.

21. Edward Wagner, "The Cost-Quality Relationship: Do We Always Get What We Pay For?" *Journal of the American Medical Association* 272, no. 24 (28 December 1994): 1951.

22. McGarvey, 45.

23. Orentlicher, "Managed Care," 22.

24. See McGarvey, 45. Also see Orentlicher, "Managed Care," 21.

25. E. Haavi Morreim, *Balancing Act: The New Medical Ethics of Medicine's New Economics* (Dordrecht, The Netherlands: Kluwer Academic Publishers, 1991).

26. J. D. Kleine, "Triumph of the Market," *Barron's*, 24 October 1994, 59.

27. Malik M. Hasan, "Let's End the Non-Profit Charade," *New England Journal of Medicine* 334, no. 16 (18 April 1996): 1055–1056.

28. Erik Larson, "The Soul of an HMO," *Time*, 22 January 1996, 49.

29. David Segal, "Health Care Costs Hit Milestone," *Washington Post*, 28 September 1995, D13.

30. Lloyd M. Kreiger, "How Managed Care Will Allow Market Forces to Solve the Problems," *New York Times*, 13 August 1995, F12 (L).

31. See Miles F. Shore and Harry Levinson, "On Business and Medicine," *New England Journal of Medicine* 313, no. 5 (1 August 1985): 319–321. Although the argument employed by these authors is on behalf of for-profit hospitals, it can be extended to apply to MCOs.

32. Cited in Linda O. Praeger, "State Licensing Boards Consider Curbing Financial Incentives," *American Medical News* 38, no. 39 (16 October 1995): 1+. Also see Kleine, 59.

33. Michael Quint, "Health Plans Are Forcing Change in the Method for Paying Doctors," *New York Times*, 5 February 1995, D5.

34. Cited in Claudia Morain, "Looking for More Controls on Managed Care in California," *American Medical News* 38, no. 18 (8 May 1995): 5.

35. Julie Kosterlitz, "Unmanaged Care?" *National Journal* (10 December 1994): 2907.

36. See Hasan, 1057–1059.

37. Ronald E. Cann, "Managed Care, Mental Health, and the Marketplace," Letter to the Editor, *Journal of the American Medical Association* 271, no. 8 (24 February 1994): 587.

38. Robert Moffit, "Personal Freedom and Responsibility: The Ethical Foundations of a Market-Based Health Care Reform System," *Journal of Medicine and Philosophy* 19, no. 5 (October 1994): 471–480.

39. Uwe Reinhardt, "Managed Competition in Health Care Reform: Just Another American Dream or the Perfect Solution?" *Journal of Law, Medicine & Ethics* 22, no. 2 (Summer 1994): 106–120.

40. Robert Tenery Jr., "Competition May Ensure Quality in Managed Care," *American Medical News* 38, no. 17 (1 May 1995): 25–26.

41. See Ron Winslow, "Employer Costs Slip As Workers Shift to HMO's," *Wall Street Journal*, 14 February 1995, A3; and Ron Stodghill et al., "Sudden Illness," *Business Week*, 8 May 1995, 32.

42. David R. Olmos, "California Care Scores Poorly in Quality Review," *Los Angeles Times*, 5 October 1995, D6.

43. H. Tristam Engelhardt, Jr., and Michael A. Rie, "Morality for the Emerging Medical Industrial Complex," *New England Journal of Medicine* 319, no. 16 (20 October 1988): 1086.

44. Mark H. Waymack, "Health Care as a Business: The Ethic of Hippocrates Versus the Ethic of Managed Care," *Business and Professional Ethics Journal* 9, nos. 3&4 (1990): 74–75.

45. Waymack, 76.

46. Jim Schachter, "Insured People Satisfied with Medical Care," *Los Angeles Times*, 28 August 1995, A13.

47. Cited in Engelhardt and Rie, 1088.

48. H. S. Luft, and R. H. Miller, "Patient Selection in a Competitive Health System," *Health Affairs* 7, no. 3 (1988): 97–119, cited in John K. Inglehart, "The American Health Care System: Managed Care," *New England Journal of Medicine* 327, no. 10 (3 September 1992): 746.

49. Engelhardt and Rie, 1086.

50. "An Anti-Patient Act," *New York Times*, 31 May 1995, A20 (L). See also Janice Castro, "Who Owns the Patient Anyway?" *Time*, 18 July 1994, 38–40.

51. George Anders and Laura Johannes, "Doctors Are Losing a Lobbying Battle to HMO's," *Wall Street Journal*, 15 May 1995, B1+.

52. Cited in Kosterlitz, 2907.

53. See Phillip M. Nudelman and Linda M. Andrews, "The 'Value Added' of Not-for-Profit Health Plans," *New England Journal of Medicine* 334, no. 16 (18 April 1995): 1058–1059.

54. Kate T. Christensen, "Ethically Important Distinctions among Managed Care Organizations," *Journal of Law, Medicine & Ethics* 23 (1995): 223–229.

55. See Oliver Goldsmith, "HMO Revolution in California," Letter to the Editor, *Los Angeles Times*, 6 September 1995, B8. Goldsmith, medical director of the Southern California Kaiser-Permanente Group, admonishes the *Times* for missing this distinction in a recent series on health maintenance organizations.

56. Carolyn M. Clancy and Howard Brody, "Managed Care: Jekyll or Hyde?" *Journal of the American Medical Association* 273, no. 4 (25 January 1995): 338–339.

57. Arnold Relman, "What Market Values Are Doing to Medicine," *Atlantic Monthly*, March 1992, 106.

58. Arnold Relman, cited in Susan Wolf, "Health Care Reform and the Future of Physician Ethics," *Hastings Center Report* 24, no. 2 (1994): 33.

59. Clancy and Brody, "Managed Care: Jekyll or Hyde?" 338–339.

60. This will be discussed in some detail in chapter 6. A high ratio is usually interpreted as more favorable to patients.

61. See Joseph Sullivan, "Officials Scrutinizing Doctor Bonuses in Managed Care Plans," *New York Times*, 21 September 1995, B6(L).

62. See Nudelman and Andrews.

63. Cardinal Joseph Bernardin, "The Case for Not-for-Profit Health Care," speech delivered at the Harvard Business School Club of Chicago, 12 January 1995.

64. Clancy and Brody, "Managed Care: Jekyll or Hyde?" 338–339. Also see Ezekial J. Emanuel and Nancy Neveloff Dubler, Reply to Letters to the

Editor, *Journal of the American Medical Association* 274, no. 8 (23/30 August 1995): 610.

65. Arnold S. Relman, "Medical Practice under the Clinton Reforms: Avoiding Domination by Big Business," *New England Journal of Medicine* 329, no. 21 (18 November 1993): 1574.

66. See Castro, 38–40.

67. See Brian McCormick, "Law Thwarts Physician Networks," *American Medical News* 38, no. 33 (4 September 1995): 1. Also see Cindy Skrzycki, "Doctors Lobby Congress in Tug of War over Patients," *Washington Post*, 6 October 1995, F1.

68. David R. Olmos, "HMO's Shut Out of Latest Health Care Trend," *Los Angeles Times*, 27 October 1996, A1.

69. Carolyn M. Clancy and Howard Brody, Reply to Letters to the Editor, *Journal of the American Medical Association* 274, no. 8 (23/30 August 1995): 611.

70. See Nancy Jecker, "Business Ethics and the Ethics of Managed Care," *Trends in Health Care, Law & Ethics* 10, no. 1/2 (Winter/Spring 1995): 55.

71. See Castro, 40.

72. See Alain C. Enthoven and Richard Kronick, "A Consumer Choice Plan for the 1990's: Universal Health Insurance in a System Designed to Promote Quality and Economy," *New England Journal of Medicine* 320 (1988): 29–37.

73. Michael Stoker, "The Ticket to Better Managed Care," *New York Times*, 28 October 1995, 21(L)

Four FEE-FOR-SERVICE MEDICINE

1. Giles Scofield, "Mangled Care," *Trends in Health Care, Law & Ethics* 10, no. 1/2 (Winter/Spring 1995): 50.

2. See Sam Sugar, Letter to the Editor, *New England Journal of Medicine* 333, no. 18 (2 November 1995): 1220.

3. Milton Friedman, "The Social Responsibility of Business Is to Increase Its Profits," *New York Times Magazine*, 13 September 1970, 32–33, 122–126.

4. Wendy K. Mariner, "Business vs. Medical Ethics: Conflicting Standards for Managed Care," *Journal of Law, Medicine & Ethics* 23 (1995): 238.

5. See Uwe Reinhardt in Arnold Relman and Uwe Reinhardt, "An Exchange on For-Profit Health Care," Institute of Medicine, *For-Profit Enterprise in Health Care* (Washington D.C.: National Academy Press, 1986), 211.

6. See Arnold Relman's statement in Relman and Reinhardt, 210. Although Relman is not what I have categorized as a Patient-Centered Purist, his point is consistent with the views of those who fit under this type.

7. See Reinhardt, in Relman and Reinhardt, 211–212. Also see Andrew C. Wicks, "Albert Schweitzer or Ivan Boesky? Why We Should Reject the Dichotomy between Medicine and Business," *Journal of Business Ethics* 14, no. 5 (May 1995): 339–351.

8. See Dan W. Brock and Allen E. Buchanan, "The Profit Motive in Medicine," *Journal of Medicine and Philosophy* 12 (1987): 1–35; Dan Brock, "Medicine and Business: An Unhealthy Mix?" *Business and Professional Ethics Journal*, 9, nos. 3&4 (1990): 21–37; Wicks, "Albert Schweitzer or Ivan Boesky?" 339–351; and Miles F. Shore and Harry Levinson, "On Business and Medicine," *New England Journal of Medicine* 313, no. 5 (1 August 1985): 319–321.

9. See for example, Robert Solomon, *Ethics and Excellence: Cooperation and Integrity in Business* (New York: Oxford University Press, 1992).

10. My point in raising the existence of these models at this juncture is to show that business does not always run along the lines of the wealth maximization model. Furthermore, there is no universal agreement within the business ethics literature that it should. I will elaborate upon this point in detail in chapter 5.

11. See Shore and Levinson for remarks about a longer-term view of business. As I will make clear in a later chapter, the assumption that ethics has to be devoid of self-interest is a false and unrealistic one.

12. David Orentlicher, "Managed Care and the Threat to the Patient-Physician Relationship," *Trends in Health Care, Law & Ethics* 10, no. 1/2 (Winter/Spring 1995): 21.

13. *American Journal of Public Health*, October 1994, and CDC/NCHS Advance Data No. 254 (3 August 1994), both cited in Michael McGarvey, "The Case for Managed Care," *Trends in Health Care, Law & Ethics* 10, no. 1/2 (Winter/Spring 1995): 46.

14. Ron Stodghill II et al., "Sudden Illness: Managed Care Faces a Harsh New Reality," *Business Week*, 8 May 1995, 32–33.

15. David Segal, "Health Care Costs Hit Milestone," *Washington Post*, 28 September 1995, D13.

16. See Jeff Goldsmith et al., "Managed Care Comes of Age," *Healthcare Forum Journal* (September/October 1995): 14–24; and Robert M. Tenery, Jr., "Competition May Ensure Quality in Managed Care," *American Medical News* 38, (1 May 1995): 25–26.

17. Julie Kosterlitz, "Unmanaged Care?" *National Journal* (10 December 1994): 2907.

18. Ron Winslow, "Big Buyers of Health Care Unite to Rate HMO's," *Wall Street Journal*, 3 July 1995, A3.

19. Michael A. Hiltzik, "Drawing the Line: An HMO Dilemma," *Los Angeles Times*, 17 January 1996, A1.

20. See George Rainbolt, "Competition and the Patient-Centered Ethic," *Journal of Medicine and Philosophy* 12 (1987): 85–99; and Uwe Reinhardt in Relman and Reinhardt, 210–216.

21. Reinhardt, in Relman and Reinhardt, 215.

22. See G. J. Agich, "Medicine as a Business and Profession," *Theoretical Medicine* 11 (1990): 311–324, cited in Jecker, "Managed Competition and Managed Care: What Are the Ethical Issues?" *Clinics in Geriatric Medicine* 10, no. 3 (August 1994): 534.

23. Bettijane Levine, "He Might Have the Cure for Medicine's Ills," *Los Angeles Times*, 18 July 1995, E6.

24. David R. Olmos and Michael Hiltzik, "Doctors Authority, Pay Dwindle under HMO's," *Los Angeles Times*, 29 August 1995, A1.

25. Reinhardt, in Relman and Reinhardt, 212.

26. Edward B. Hirshfield, "Should Ethical and Legal Standards for Physicians Be Changed to Accommodate New Models of Rationing Health Care?" *University of Pennsylvania Law Review* 140, no. 1755 (1992): 1840.

27. Janice Castro, "Who Owns the Patient Anyway?" *Time*, 18 July 1994, 38–40.

28. See Marc A. Rodwin, *Money, Medicine and Morals* (New York: Oxford University Press, 1993).

29. See Edmund D. Pellegrino, "Words Can Hurt You: Some Reflections on the Metaphors of Managed Care," First Annual Nicholas Pisano Lecture, *Journal of the American Board of Family Practice* 7, no. 6 (November–December 1994): 508; and Ruth Macklin, "The Ethics of

Managed Care," *Trends in Health Care, Law & Ethics* 10, no. 1/2 (Winter/Spring 1995): 63–66.

30. See Rodwin, *Money, Medicine and Morals*, and Dan Brock, "Medicine and Business: An Unhealthy Mix?"

31. See Rodwin, *Money, Medicine and Morals*.

32. John Wennberg, "Analysis of Nationwide Medicare Statistics," presented at meeting of American College of Cardiology, March 1995, and Norman Kato, "Variations in Managed Care Among Small Areas," *Scientific American* (April 1982): 120–134, both cited in McGarvey, 45.

33. Brock and Buchanan, 24.

34. Reinhardt, in Relman and Reinhardt, 212.

35. See Wicks, "Albert Schweitzer or Ivan Boesky?" 342; and Patricia Werhane, "The Ethics of Health Care as a Business," *Business and Professional Ethics Journal* 9, nos. 3&4 (Fall–Winter 1990): 7–20.

36. Reinhardt, in Relman and Reinhardt, 211–212.

37. Paul Starr (1992), cited in Brock and Buchanan, 24.

38. Scofield, 48.

39. Ibid. Also see Jecker, "Managed Competition and Managed Care," 530–532.

40. Paul Fieldstein, "The Political Economy of Health Care," in *Health Economics* (New York: John Wiley and Sons, 1979), cited in Reinhardt, in Relman and Reinhardt, 214.

41. See "An Anti-Patient Act," *New York Times*, 31 May 1995, A20(L).

42. John K. Inglehart, "The Struggle between Managed Care and Fee-for-Service Practice," *New England Journal of Medicine* 331, no. 1 (7 July 1994): 66.

43. Robert A. Rosenblatt and Edwin Chen, "AMA Backs GOP Medicare Plan," *Los Angeles Times*, 11 October 1995, A1+.

44. See Robert A. Rosenblatt, "Doctors Prescribe Medicare HMO's as Panacea for Ailing Bottom Lines," *Los Angeles Times*, 25 November 1995, A29.

45. Randall J. Lewis, Letter to the Editor, *New England Journal of Medicine* 333, no. 18 (2 November 1995): 1220.

46. Jeff McCombs, "Health Care," Letter to the Editor, *Los Angeles Times*, 8 January 1996, B4.

47. See Michael S. Broder, "In Health Care, We Cannot Have It All," *Los Angeles Times*, 27 December 1995, B9. Also see McCombs, B4.

48. See Goldsmith et al.

49. Goldsmith et al., 24.

50. Michael Quint, "Health Plans Are Forcing Change in the Method for Paying Doctors," *New York Times*, 5 February 1995, D5.

51. See Mark R. Chassin, "The Missing Ingredient in Health Reform: Quality of Care" *Journal of the American Medical Association* 270, no. 3 (21 July 1993): 377–378; and Jerome P. Kassirer, "The Quality of Care and the Quality of Measuring It," *New England Journal of Medicine* 329, no. 17 (21 October 1993): 1263–1265.

52. John E. Ware et al., "Differences in 4-Year Health Outcomes for Elderly and Poor, Chronically Ill Patients Treated in HMO and Fee-for-Service Systems: Results from the Medical Outcomes Study," *Journal of the American Medical Association* 276, no. 13 (2 October 1996): 1039–1047.

53. Dana Gelb Safran et al., "Primary Care Performance in Fee-for-Service and Prepaid Health Care Systems," *Journal of the American Medical Association* 271, no. 20 (25 May 1994): 1579–1586.

54. The Virginia study is cited in George W. Rilmer and Richard D. Morrison, "The Ethical Impacts of Managed Care," *Journal of Business Ethics* 12, no. 6 (June 1993): 493–501.

55. Dolores G. Clement et al., "Access and Outcomes of Elderly Patients Enrolled in Managed Care," *Journal of the American Medical Association* 271, no. 19 (18 May 1994): 1487–1492.

56. *Annals of Internal Medicine*, 5 January 1987, cited in McGarvey, 46.

57. Barbara Starfield et al., "Cost vs. Quality in Different Types of Primary Care Settings," *Journal of the American Medical Association* 272, no. 24 (28 December 1994): 1903.

58. Institute of Medicine, "Controlling Costs and Changing Patient Care? The Role of Utilization Management" (Washington D.C.: National Academy Press, 1989), cited in Rilmer and Morrison, 497.

59. Sheldon Greenfield et al., "Outcomes of Patients with Hypertension and Non-Insulin-Dependent Diabetes Mellitus Treated by Different Systems and Specialties: Results from the Medical Outcomes Study," *Journal of the American Medical Association* 274 (8 November 1995): 1436–1474, cited in Ware et al.

60. P. Braveman et al., "Insurance-Related Differences in the Risk of Ruptured Appendix," *New England Journal of Medicine* 331 (1994): 444–449, cited in Arnold S. Relman, "What About Managed Care?" *New England Journal of Medicine* 331, no. 7 (18 August 1994): 471–472.

61. Relman, "What About Managed Care?" 472.

62. Carolyn M. Clancy and Howard Brody, Reply to Letters to the Editor, *Journal of the American Medical Association* 274, no. 8 (23/30 August 1995): 611.

63. Clancy and Brody, Reply to Letters to the Editor, 611.

64. Jecker, "Managed Competition and Managed Care," 535.

65. Ibid., 535–536.

66. M. Stanton Evans et al., "The Trouble with HMO's," *Consumers' Research*, July 1994, 12.

67. CBO study, cited in Evans et al., 12, and in Amy K. Taylor et al., "Who Belongs to HMO's: A Comparison of Fee-for-Service versus HMO Enrollees," *Medical Care Research and Review* 52, no. 3 (September 1995): 389–408.

68. See Goldsmith et al., 22.

69. Sandra Johnson, "Managed Care as Regulation: Functional Ethics for a Regulated Environment," *Journal of Law, Medicine & Ethics* 23 (1995): 268.

70. Alan L. Hillman, Pete Welch and Mark V. Pauly, "Contractual Arrangements between HMO's and Primary Care Physicians: Three-Tiered HMO's and Risk Pools," *Medical Care* 30, no. 2 (February 1992): 136–148.

71. Johnson, 268.

72. Quint, "Health Plans Are Forcing Change," A1.

73. John LaPuma, Letter to the Editor, *Journal of the American Medical Association* 274, no. 8 (23/30 August 1995): 610.

74. Clancy and Brody, Reply to Letters to the Editor, 611.

Five ALTERNATIVE REFORM PROPOSALS

1. David E. Kim, Letter to the Editor, *New England Journal of Medicine* 333, no. 18 (2 November 1995): 1220.

2. John C. Goodman, "A Plan to Empower Patients," *Wall Street Journal*, 2 May 1995, A24.

3. Howard Stock, Letter to the Editor, *Journal of the American Medical Association* 271, no. 8 (23 February 1994): 588.

4. Kenneth E. Thorpe, "Medical Savings Accounts: Design and Policy Issues," *Health Affairs* 14, no. 3 (1995): 258.

5. See Bruce Ramsey, "Medical Savings Accounts Turn Out to Be Hard Sell," *Seattle Post-Intelligencer* (24 September 1997): E1.

6. Uwe Reinhardt, "Managed Competition in Health Reform: Just Another American Dream, or the Perfect Solution?" *Journal of Law, Medicine & Ethics* 22, no. 2 (Summer 1994): 107. Reinhardt cites the source of this data as the Medstat Corporation of Ann Arbor, Michigan.

7. Thorpe, 258.

8. Goodman, "A Plan to Empower Patients," A24.

9. David Orentlicher, "Managed Care and the Threat to the Patient-Physician Relationship," *Trends in Health Care, Law & Ethics* 10, no. 1/2 (Winter/Spring 1995): 20–21.

10. Ibid.

11. Edward B. Hirshfield, "Should Ethical and Legal Standards for Physicians Be Changed to Accommodate New Models for Rationing Health Care?" *University of Pennsylvania Law Review* 140 (1992):1818–1819.

12. Arthur Caplan, "Can Money and Morality Mix in Medicine?" *Academic Emergency Medicine* 1, no. 1 (January/February 1994): 77.

13. David Mechanic, "Professional Judgment and the Rationing of Health Care," *University of Pennsylvania Law Review* 140 (1992): 1723.

14. Orentlicher, "Managed Care," 20.

15. E. Haavi Morreim, "Cost Containment: Challenging Fidelity and Justice," *Hastings Center Report* (December 1988): 22.

16. Ibid.

17. Orentlicher, "Managed Care," 20.

18. Caplan, 78–79.

19. David C. Hadorn, "Setting Health Care Priorities in Oregon: Effectiveness Meets the Rule of Rescue," *Journal of the American Medical Association* 265 (1991): 2218–2219, cited in Mechanic, 1744.

20. See Carolyn M. Clancy and Howard Brody, Reply to Letters to the Editor, *Journal of the American Medical Association* 274, no. 8 (23/30 August 1995): 611.

21. Orentlicher, "Managed Care," 20.

22. See Morreim, "Cost Containment," 22; and Mechanic, 1727–1728.

23. Orentlicher, "Managed Care," 20.

24. Mechanic, 1746.

25. David C. Thomasma, "The Ethics of Managed Care and Cost Control," *Trends in Health Care, Law & Ethics* 10, no. 1/2 (Winter/Spring 1995): 33.

26. David S. Broder, "Managed Care Savings Seen," *Washington Post*, 12 May 1994, A9.

27. See Wendy K. Mariner, "Business vs. Medical Ethics: Conflicting Standards for Managed Care," *Journal of Law, Medicine & Ethics* 23 (1995): 245–246, note 64; and Michael Quint, "Health Plans Are Forcing Change in the Method for Paying Doctors," *New York Times*, 5 February 1995, D5.

Six   THE ETHICAL IMPORTANCE OF
       THE NON-PROFIT DISTINCTION

1. See Edmund Pellegrino, "Interests, Obligations, and Justice: Some Notes toward an Ethic of Managed Care," *Journal of Clinical Ethics* 6 (1995): 316.

2. Kate T. Christensen, "Ethically Important Distinctions among Managed Care Organizations," *Journal of Law, Medicine & Ethics* 23 (1995): 223; and Pellegrino, "Interests, Obligations, and Justice," 316.

3. A. Yarmolinsky, "Supporting the Patient," *New England Journal of Medicine* 332 (1995): 602–603, cited in Jerome P. Kassirer, "Managed Care and the Morality of the Marketplace," *New England Journal of Medicine* 331, no. 1 (6 July 1995): 51.

4. Cardinal Joseph Bernardin, "The Case for Not-for-Profit Health Care," speech delivered at the Harvard Business School Club of Chicago, 12 January 1995.

5. Christensen, 226.

6. Carolyn M. Clancy and Howard Brody, "Managed Care: Jekyll or Hyde?" *Journal of the American Medical Association* 273, no. 4 (25 January 1995): 339.

7. Phillip M. Nudelman and Linda M. Andrews, "The 'Value-Added' of Not-for-Profit Health Plans," *New England Journal of Medicine* 334, no. 18 (18 April 1996): 1057.

8. Frederick R. Abrams, "Caring for the Sick: An Emerging Industrial By-Product," *Journal of the American Medical Association* 255, no. 7 (21 February 1986): 937–938.

9. Douglas P. Shuit, "State Medical Association to Cite High Cost of Private Health Plans," *Los Angeles Times*, 18 April 1995, A3.

10. See Dan W. Brock and Allen E. Buchanan, "The Profit Motive in Medicine," *Journal of Medicine and Philosophy* 12 (1987): 1–35. Although these authors support for-profit enterprises in medicine, they give a detailed discussion of cost-shifting/cross-subsidization practices.

11. Brock and Buchanan, 11–12.

12. Ibid., 10.

13. W. G. Manning et al., "Health Insurance and the Demand for Health Care," *American Economic Review* (June 1987): 251–277, cited in Kenneth Thorpe, "Medical Savings Accounts Design and Policy Issues," *Health Affairs* 14, no. 3 (1995): 254–259. As noted earlier, these studies suggest that moving from "free" care to a fee-for-service plan with a 25 percent copayment could reduce total outlays by 23 percent.

14. See, for example, Kassirer, "Managed Care," 52.

15. Uwe Reinhardt, in Arnold Relman and Uwe Reinhardt, "An Exchange on For-Profit Health Care," Institute of Medicine, *For-Profit Enterprise in Health Care* (Washington, D.C.: National Academy Press, 1986), 213.

16. Ibid., 214.

17. See David C. Thomasma, "The Ethics of Managed Care and Cost Control," *Trends in Health Care, Law & Ethics* 10, no. 1/2 (Winter/Spring 1995): 33; and James Flannigan, "The Changing State of Managed Care," *Los Angeles Times*, 23 June 1996, D1.

18. Howard Wolinsky, "Ethics in Managed Care," *The Lancet* 345 (10 June 1995): 1499.

19. E. Haavi Morreim, "Moral Justice and Legal Justice in Managed Care: The Ascent of Contributory Justice," *Journal of Law, Medicine & Ethics* 23 (1995): 253.

20. Nudelman and Andrews, 1057.

21. These positive changes include expanded options to see out-of-network physicians and the use of specialists without gatekeeper referral; also, some insurers, such as Health Net, now send reviews

for experimental treatment decisions to independent outside agencies.

22. Norman Daniels, "The Profit Motive and the Moral Assessment of Health Care Institutions," *Business and Professional Ethics Journal* 10, no. 2 (Summer 1991): 6.

23. Philip Boyle, "Business Ethics in Ethics Committees?" *Hastings Center Report* (September/October 1990): 37.

24. Brock and Buchanan, 6.

25. Nudelman and Andrews, 1059.

26. See for example, The Catholic Health Association, "The Values Motivating the CHA Working Proposal for Systematic Healthcare Reform," in *Setting Relationships Right: A Working Proposal For Systematic Health Care Reform* (Washington, D.C.: The Catholic Health Association, 1992), 2.

27. Daniels, 6.

28. Ibid.

29. Eve Kerr et al., "Managed Care and Capitation in California: How Do Physicians at Financial Risk Control Their Own Utilization?" *Annals of Internal Medicine* 123 (1995): 500–504.

30. In addition to the controversy surrounding the early release of mothers and their newborns, Kaiser has been involved in at least two other widely publicized controversies. In what is widely believed to be the first effort of its kind, the organization announced plans to pay bonuses to *nurses* who helped to reduce costs in its treatment facilities, generating wide public protest. For a more detailed discussion of this controversy, see David Olmos, "Kaiser Seeking to Pay Bonuses to Nurses Who Help Cut Costs," *Los Angeles Times*, 22 December 1995, D1. In another situation, Kaiser acted in a manner consistent with accusations that for-profit organizations define the term "experimental" so broadly in decisions that they exclude legitimate treatments. Kaiser was recently sued for contributing to the death of a patient by withholding a treatment for cancer, similar to the case involving Christy deMeurers and her insurer, Health Net, which denied a bone marrow transplant. The suit is pending because it was preempted by ERISA laws and was removed from the state court jurisdiction. For a more detailed account of this case, see Michael Hiltzik, "Supreme Court Won't Allow State Suit in Case," *Los Angeles Times*, 16 May 1995, D1.

31. See Nudelman and Andrews, 1057, and Wolinsky, 1499, quoting Arnold Relman.

32. U.S. Health Care is mentioned in Alan L. Hillman and Neil Goldfarb, "Exemplary Quality Improvement Programs in HMO's," *Journal of Quality Improvement* 21 (September 1995): 457–464; and in R. W. Morrow, A. D. Gooding, and C. Clark, "Improving Physicians' Preventative Health Care Behavior through Peer Review and Financial Incentives," *Archives of Family Medicine* 4 (1995): 165–169, cited in Arthur Leibowitz, Nicholas A. Hanchak, and Neil Schlackman, "Corporate Managed Care," *New England Journal of Medicine* 334, no. 16 (18 April 1996): 1060.

33. Steffie Woolhandler and David Himmelstein, Letter to the Editor, *New England Journal of Medicine* 334, no. 16 (18 April 1996): 1062.

34. See Christensen, 223; and Alan Mittermaier, "Give Your HMO a Thorough Annual Checkup," *Wall Street Journal*, 9 October 1995, A12(E).

35. Christensen, 223.

36. Wolinsky, 1499.

37. Christensen, 223.

38. See "How HMO Expenses Break Down," *Los Angeles Times*, 15 February 1996, D2, citing the California Medical Association, *1994–95 Knox-Keene Health Plan Expenditures Summary*, Sacramento, California, February 1996; and the *1995–96 Knox-Keene Health Plan Expenditures Summary*, February 1997; see also Christensen, 223, citing Steve Thompson and Zabrae Valentine, "The Profiteering of HMO's," *California Physician* (July 1994): 8–34.

39. California Medical Association, *1994–95 Knox-Keene Health Plan Expenditures Summary*, and *1995–96 Knox-Keene Health Plan Expenditures Summary*.

40. California Medical Association, *1994–95 Summary*, 4.

41. This size distinction was used by the California Management Association in the *Knox-Keene Summary, 1994–95* and *1995–96* editions.

42. California Medical Association, *1995–96 Summary*, 10–11.

43. California Medical Association, *1994–95 Summary*, 4–8, and *1995–96 Summary*, 10–11.

44. California Medical Association, *1994–95 Summary*, 9–10, and *1995–96 Summary*, 8–9.

45. California Medical Association, *1995–96 Summary*, 8–9.

46. Ibid., "Executive Summary", ii, note 2.

47. Ibid., note 4. In addition to these errors, the 1995–96 version of the report also acknowledges that earlier versions failed to account for the differences between investment income versus income from premium and operating sources. See note 1.

48. See Alain C. Enthoven and Richard Kronick, "Universal Health Insurance through Incentives Reform," *Journal of the American Medical Association* 265, no. 19 (15 May 1991): 2532–2536.

49. The latest version of the report acknowledges that MLRs "do not directly measure quality of care." See California Medical Association, *1995–96 Summary*, "Executive Summary," ii, note 4.

50. David R. Olmos, "Members Like Small HMO's Best, Poll Says," *Los Angeles Times*, 12 September 1996, D2.

51. Nudelman and Andrews, 1057.

52. Brock and Buchanan, 4.

53. Uwe Reinhardt, in Relman and Reinhardt, 212–213.

54. Ibid., 211.

55. Ibid.

Seven THE MORAL VIABILITY OF FOR-PROFIT ORGANIZATIONS

1. Malik M. Hasan, "Let's End the Non-Profit Charade," *New England Journal of Medicine* 334, no. 16 (18 April 1996): 1055.

2. J. D. Kleinke, "Triumph of the Market," *Barron's*, 24 October 1994, 59.

3. See Julie Kosterlitz, "Unmanaged Care?" *National Journal* (10 December 1994): 2907; and Charles Schmidt Jr., "Managed Care Faces Stinging Backlash," *Best's Review* (November 1995): 22–23.

4. Hasan, 1056.

5. Hasan, 1055–1057.

6. See for example, Ronald E. Cann, "Managed Care, Mental Health, and the Marketplace," Letter to the Editor, *Journal of the American Medical Association* 271, no. 8 (23 February 1994): 587.

7. Kleinke, 59.

8. See Kosterlitz, 2904, citing Susan Pisano.

9. Westcott Price III, "Managed Care Now; It Works," *Los Angeles Times*, 14 March 1995, B7.

10. Brian Gould and Eugene D. Hill, Letter to the Editor, *Journal of the American Medical Association* 271, no. 8 (23 February 1994): 588.

11. Ibid.

12. H. Tristam Engelhardt Jr. and Michael A. Rie, "Morality for the Emerging Medical Industrial Complex," *New England Journal of Medicine* 319, no. 16 (20 October 1988): 1086.

13. Mark H. Waymack, "Health Care as a Business: The Ethic of Hippocrates versus the Ethic of Managed Care," *Business and Professional Ethics Journal* 9, nos. 3&4 (1990): 74–75.

14. See Kosterlitz, 2905; and Jim Schachter, "Insured People Satisfied with Medical Care," *Los Angeles Times*, 28 August 1995, A1.

15. Joel Cantor et al., "Private Employer-Based Health Insurance in Ten States," *Health Affairs* 14, no. 2 (1995): 199–211, cited in Wendy K. Mariner, "Business vs. Medical Ethics: Conflicting Standards for Managed Care," *Journal of Law, Medicine & Ethics* 23 (1995): 240.

16. Deborah Chollet, "Employer-Based Health Insurance in a Changing Work Force," *Health Affairs* 13, no. 1 (1994): 327–336, cited in Mariner, 240.

17. As I noted in chapter 1, ERISA laws preempt many state-level legal remedies which patients may otherwise have as recourse against managed care organizations. See the section entitled "The Current Legal Environment" in chapter 1 for a further discussion.

18. Patricia H. Werhane, *Adam Smith and His Legacy for Modern Capitalism* (New York: Oxford University Press, 1991).

19. Dan Brock and Allen Buchanan mention this "free-rider" problem with respect to providing care for the indigent. See Brock and Buchanan, "The Profit Motive in Medicine," *Journal of Medicine and Philosophy* 12 (1987): 14.

20. Erik Larson, "The Soul of an HMO," *Time*, 22 January 1996, 48.

21. Steffie Woolhandler and David Himmelstein, Letter to the Editor, *New England Journal of Medicine* 334, no. 16 (18 April 1996): 1063.

22. Ron Winslow, "Employer Costs Slip as Workers Shift to HMO's," *Wall Street Journal*, 14 February 1995, A3. Also see David Segal, "Health Care Costs Hit Milestone," *Washington Post*, 28 September 1995, D13.

23. David R. Olmos and Michael A. Hiltzik, "Doctors Authority, Pay Dwindle under HMO's," *Los Angeles Times*, 29 August 1995, A1.

24. See Thomas Bodenheimer and Kevin Grumbach, "The Reconfiguration of U.S. Medicine," *Journal of the American Medical Association* 274, no. 1 (5 July 1995): 88.

25. Lloyd Kreiger, "How Managed Care Will Allow Market Forces to Solve the Problems," *New York Times*, 13 August 1995, F12(L).

26. Alan L. Hillman and Neil Goldfarb, "Exemplary Quality Improvement Programs in HMO's," *Journal of Quality Improvement* 21, no. 9 (September 1995): 457–464.

27. The model is published in N. Schlackman, "Evolution of Quality-Based Compensation Model: The Third Generation," *American Journal of Medical Quality* 8 (1993): 103–110, cited in Arthur Leibowitz et al., "Corporate Managed Care," Letter to the Editor, *New England Journal of Medicine* 334, no. 16 (18 April 1996): 1060.

28. Ron Stodghill II et al., "Sudden Illness: Managed Care Faces a Harsh New Reality," *Business Week*, 8 May 1995, 32–33.

29. See Jeff C. Goldsmith et al., "Managed Care Comes of Age," *Healthcare Forum Journal* (September/October 1995): 19–24; and Robert Tenery Jr., "Competition May Ensure Quality in Managed Care," *American Medical News* 38, no. 17 (1 May 1995): 25–26.

30. David R. Olmos, "Blue Shield, in Bold Move, Will Waive Specialist Referrals," *Los Angeles Times*, 18 June 1996, D1.

31. Examples of traditional medical ethics categories can be found in Woodstock Theological Center, *Ethical Considerations in the Business Aspects of Managed Care* (Washington, D.C.: Georgetown University Press, 1995); and Council on Ethical and Judicial Affairs, American Medical Association, "Ethical Issues in Managed Care," *Journal of the American Medical Association* 273, no. 4 (25 January 1996): 330–335. For an example of the use of a free-market oriented position, see Lester Thurow, "Medicine versus Economics," *New England Journal of Medicine* 313 (1985): 611–614, cited in Mariner, 238.

32. Mariner, 238–239.

33. Mariner and Susan Wolf note the need for *organizational* ethics that cannot be delegated to individuals. See Mariner, 238, 241; and Susan Wolf, "Health Care Reform and the Future of Physician Ethics," *Hastings Center Report* 24, no. 2 (March/April 1994): 28–41.

1. Such negative depictions of business are pervasive. Scenarios in which the corporate pursuit of profit conflicts with other social interests such as full employment, public safety, individual privacy, and a host of other moral norms have filled newspaper columns and television "news magazine" segments. On an almost weekly basis, television programs such as ABC's 20/20, Primetime Live!, NBC's Dateline, and CBS's 48 Hours feature a segment on an issue involving business vs. society. Feature-length films often utilize themes of conspiring, evil corporations. While films like *Wall Street*, *The Firm*, and *Glengarry Glen Ross* are more obvious ones, evil corporations also play ominous roles (much like the CIA or "The Company" used to play) in movies such as *The Pelican Brief*, *The Net*, and *Jerry McGuire*. The less negative, but nonetheless questionable, amoral view of business comes in the form of assumptions that financial goals are separate from moral ones. From this perspective, ethical concerns are assumed to be mere afterthoughts to economic efficiency.

2. For a more detailed description of this portrayal and a critical assessment of it, see Robert C. Solomon, "The Myth of the Profit Motive," in his *Ethics and Excellence: Cooperation and Integrity in Business* (New York: Oxford University Press, 1992): 39–47.

3. Milton Friedman, "The Social Responsibility of Business Is to Increase Its Profits," *New York Times Magazine*, 13 September 1970, 32–33, 122–126.

4. See Nancy Jecker, "Managed Competition and Managed Care: What Are the Ethical Issues?" *Clinics in Geriatric Medicine* 10, no. 3 (August 1994): 534; Andrew C. Wicks, "Albert Schweitzer or Ivan Boesky? Why We Should Reject the Dichotomy between Medicine and Business," *Journal of Business Ethics* 14, no. 5 (May 1995): 343; and Uwe Reinhardt, in Arnold Relman and Uwe Reinhardt, "An Exchange on For-Profit Health Care," in Institute of Medicine, *For-Profit Enterprise in Health Care* (Washington, D.C.: National Academy Press, 1986): 219–220.

5. Wicks, "Albert Schweitzer or Ivan Boesky?" 341, 342. Nancy Jecker and Uwe Reinhardt offer similar assessments. See Jecker, 534; and Reinhardt, in Relman and Reinhardt, 211–216.

6. See Wicks, "Albert Schweitzer or Ivan Boesky?"; and R. Edward

Freeman, "The Business Sucks Story," presidential address delivered at the annual meeting of the Society for Business Ethics, Vancouver, B.C., August 1995.

7. Patricia Werhane, "The Ethics of Health Care As a Business," *Business and Professional Ethics Journal* 9, nos. 3&4 (Fall–Winter 1990): 15. For a more comprehensive treatment of the topic, see Werhane, *Adam Smith and His Legacy for Modern Capitalism* (New York: Oxford University Press, 1991).

8. Werhane, "Ethics of Health Care as a Business," 14.

9. For a detailed discussion of the trust necessary for an efficient economy, see Francis Fukuyama, *Trust: The Social Virtues and the Creation of Prosperity* (New York: Free Press, 1995).

10. Philip Boyle, "Business Ethics in Ethics Committees?" *Hastings Center Report* (September/October 1990): 37.

11. Patricia Werhane, "The Ethics of Insider Trading," *Journal of Business Ethics* 8 (1989): 841–845.

12. See various writings by R. Edward Freeman, including "The Politics of Stakeholder Theory: Some Future Directions," *Business Ethics Quarterly* 4 (October 1994): 409–422; Michael Novak, *This Hemisphere of Liberty* (Washington, D.C.: AEI Press, 1992), 41, and his *The Spirit of Democratic Capitalism* (Lantham, Md.: Madison Books/University Press of America, 1991), 92–95; and Wicks, "Albert Schweitzer or Ivan Boesky?"

13. Novak, *This Hemisphere of Liberty*, 41; and *The Spirit of Democratic Capitalism*, 92–95.

14. R. Edward Freeman, cited in Wicks, "Albert Schweitzer or Ivan Boesky?" 344; and Andrew C. Wicks, "Overcoming the Separation Thesis: The Need for Reconsideration of Business and Society Research," *Business and Society* 35, no. 1 (March 1996): 89–118.

15. Pietra Rivoli, "Ethical Aspects of Investor Behavior," *Journal of Business Ethics* 14, no. 4 (April 1995): 265–277.

16. Wicks, "Albert Schweitzer or Ivan Boesky?" 344.

17. Ibid. Also see Novak, *The Spirit of Democratic Capitalism*, 92–95.

18. For example, various models based upon communitarianism, virtue, and reformulations of social contract theory have been proposed. See Solomon, *Ethics and Excellence*, for a virtue-oriented model; for a social contract approach, see Thomas Donaldson, "Constructing a

Social Contract for Business," in Donaldson and Werhane, eds., *Ethical Issues in Business: A Philosophical Approach,* 2nd ed. (Englewood Cliffs, N.J.: Prentice-Hall, 1983), 153–166. For a discussion of the current direction of ongoing research in integrated social contracts theory as a model for business ethics, see Thomas W. Dunfee and Thomas Donaldson, "Contractarian Business Ethics: Current Status and Next Steps," *Business Ethics Quarterly* 5, no. 2 (April 1995): 173–186.

19. Although there are some prior treatments of the subject, the seminal formulation of the stakeholder model is generally attributed to R. Edward Freeman, *Strategic Management: A Stakeholder Approach* (Boston: Pittman Publishing, 1984). A well-known formulation of the model can be found in William M. Evan and R. Edward Freeman, "A Stakeholder Theory of the Modern Corporation: Kantian Capitalism," in Tom L. Beauchamp and Norman Bowie, eds., *Ethical Theory in Business,* 3rd ed. (Englewood Cliffs, N.J.: Prentice-Hall, 1988): 97–105.

20. Evan and Freeman, 103.

21. See, for example, Thomas Donaldson and Lee E. Preston, "The Stakeholder Theory of the Corporation: Concepts, Evidence & Implications," *Academy of Management Review* 65 (1995): 65–91.

22. R. Edward Freeman, "A Stakeholder Theory of the Modern Corporation," in Tom L. Beauchamp and Norman E. Bowie, eds., *Ethical Theory and Business,* 5th ed. (Englewood Cliffs, N.J.: Prentice-Hall, 1997), 72. This article is an edited, combined version of Evan and Freeman's earlier "A Stakeholder Theory of the Modern Corporation: Kantian Capitalism" (see note 19), and R. Edward Freeman, "The Politics of Stakeholder Theory: Some Future Directions" (see note 12). For an example of one "normative core," see Brian K. Burton and Craig P. Dunn, "Feminist Ethics As Moral Grounding for Stakeholder Theory," *Business Ethics Quarterly* 6, no. 2 (April 1996): 133–147.

23. Ibid., 73. For another use of Rawls's ideas as the normative core of stakeholder theory, see Robert A. Phillips, "Stakeholder Theory and a Principle of Fairness," *Business Ethics Quarterly* 7, no. 1 (January 1997): 51–66.

24. Ibid.

25. Kenneth Goodpaster favors an approach in which duties which are "non-fiduciary" in nature but nonetheless significant are owed to stakeholders, thus preserving the special status of shareholders. See Goodpaster, "Business Ethics and Stakeholder Analysis," *Business Ethics Quarterly* 1 (January 1991): 53–73.

26. See Jon M. Shepard et al., "The Place of Business Ethics in Business: Shifting Paradigms," *Business Ethics Quarterly* 5, no. 3 (July 1995): 577–601.

27. Ibid.

28. Wicks, "Albert Schweitzer or Ivan Boesky?" 346.

29. Ibid., 347.

30. Because the model broadens the scope of social responsibility to include other stakeholders, it provides a moral framework whereby the interests of other parties can be considered without violating exclusive moral obligations to shareholders.

31. Edmund D. Pellegrino, "Interests, Obligations, and Justice: Some Notes toward an Ethic of Managed Care," *Journal of Clinical Ethics* 6, no. 4 (Winter 1995): 314.

32. Ibid., 316. Also see Kate T. Christensen, "Ethically Important Distinctions among Managed Care Organizations," *Journal of Law, Medicine & Ethics* 23 (1995): 223.

33. See Reinhardt, in Relman and Reinhardt, 214.

34. See chapter 7 for a detailed discussion of this issue.

35. Reinhardt, in Relman and Reinhardt, 211.

36. Novak, *The Spirit of Democratic Capitalism,* 95.

37. Relman, in Relman and Reinhardt, 222.

38. Ibid.

39. Dan Brock, "Medicine and Business: An Unhealthy Mix?" *Business and Professional Ethics Journal* 9, nos. 3&4 (1990): 27.

40. George W. Rainbolt, "Competition and the Patient-Centered Ethic," *Journal of Medicine and Philosophy* 12 (1987): 90.

41. There are also many commentators who argue that business ought to be cast in more professional terms. See for example, Michael Novak, *Business as a Calling* (New York: Free Press, 1996); and Joshua D. Margolis, "Casting Business As a Profession," paper presented at the 1996 annual meeting of the Society for Business Ethics, Quebec City, August 1996.

42. Evan and Freeman, 100.

43. Andrew C. Wicks, "The Business Ethics Movement: Where Are We Headed and What Can We Learn from Our Colleagues in Bioethics?" *Business Ethics Quarterly* 5, no. 3 (1995): 608.

44. Mariner, 238.

45. William Shaw and Vincent Barry, "Corporations," in *Moral Issues in Business*, 5th ed. (Belmont, Calif.: Wadsworth Publishing, 1992), 202–209.

46. Mariner, 238.

47. See Shaw and Barry for a more comprehensive overview of this debate.

48. Manuel Velasquez, "Why Corporations Are Not Morally Responsible for Anything They Do," *Business & Professional Ethics Journal* 2 (Spring 1983): 8, cited in Shaw and Barry, 208.

49. H. R. Smith and Archie B. Carroll, "Organizational Ethics: A Stacked Deck," *Journal of Business Ethics* 3 (1984): 95–100.

50. Peter French, "The Corporation As a Moral Person," *American Philosophical Quarterly* 3 (1979): 207–215.

51. Donaldson, "Constructing a Social Contract for Business," 153–166. For a discussion of the current direction of ongoing research in integrated social contract theory as a model for business ethics, see Dunfee and Donaldson, "Contractarian Business Ethics."

52. On recent cases involving Sears Auto Centers and MetLife, see Kevin Kelly and Eric Schine, "How Did Sears Blow This Gasket?" *Business Week*, 29 June 1992, 38; and Greg Steinmetz, "Metlife Probed in Several States for Sales Tactics," *Wall Street Journal*, Eastern ed., 6 January 1994, 81.

53. Lynne Sharp Paine, "Managing for Organizational Integrity," *Harvard Business Review* (March–April 1994): 106–117.

54. The debate over the preservation of forest land for the Spotted Owl is a good example of a situation involving the problem of stakeholder adjudication. For a detailed discussion of this problem, see Dunfee and Donaldson, "Contractarian Business Ethics: Current Status and Next Steps," 175.

55. See Mariner, 239. Although Mariner uses a rather narrow interpretation of business in her critique, she gives this example in the context of an organization which she believes to have a fairly enlightened ethical code.

56. Werhane, "The Ethics of Health Care as a Business," 15–17, and Wicks, "Albert Schweitzer or Ivan Boesky?" 344.

57. Wicks, "Albert Schweitzer or Ivan Boesky?" 344–345.

58. Ibid., 347.

59. Werhane, "The Ethics of Health Care as a Business," 17.

60. See Phillips, "Stakeholder Theory and a Principle of Fairness."

61. Sandra Johnson, "Managed Care as Regulation: Functional Ethics for a Regulated Environment," *Journal of Law, Medicine & Ethics* 23 (1995): 266–272.

62. Jecker, "Managed Competition and Managed Care," 534.

Nine STAKEHOLDER RESPONSIBILITIES IN
THE NEW HEALTH CARE ENVIRONMENT

1. See Susan Wolf, "Health Care Reform and The Future of Physician Ethics," *Hastings Center Report* 24, no. 2 (1994): 28–41; and Ruth Macklin, *Enemies of Patients* (New York: Oxford University Press, 1993).

2. See Wolf, "Health Care Reform and the Future of Physician Ethics"; E. Haavi Morreim, *Balancing Act* (Dordrecht, The Netherlands: Kluwer Academic Publishers, 1991); and Ruth Macklin, *Enemies of Patients*.

3. Although there is little available evidence about the prevalence of practices such as gag orders, and spokespersons for these organizations deny their existence, anecdotal evidence from physicians abounds that they are used. See Robert A. Rosenblatt, "Doctors, HMO's Clash at Hearing 'Gag Rules'," *Los Angeles Times*, 31 May 1996, A1.

4. Examples of disclosure requirements can be found in industrial products, food packaging, and real estate transactions.

5. Susan Wolf notes that bioethics as a whole has no theory of process and is sorely in need of one. See Susan Wolf, "Toward a Theory of Process," *Law, Medicine & Health Care* (1992): 278–290; and "Health Care Reform and the Future of Physician Ethics," 38.

6. An example is the Health Plan Employer Information Data Set (HEIDS). See Bruce C. Vladeck, "Managed Care and Quality," *Journal of the American Medical Association* 273, no. 19 (17 May 1995): 1483.

7. See Mark R. Chassin, "The Missing Ingredient in Health Reform: Quality of Care," *Journal of the American Medical Association* 270, no. 3 (21 July 1993): 377–378.

8. Jerome P. Kassirer, "The Quality of Care and the Quality of Measur-

ing It," *New England Journal of Medicine* 329, no. 17 (31 October 1993): 1263–1264.

9. David Orentlicher, "Managed Care and the Threat to the Patient-Physician Relationship," *Trends in Health Care, Law & Ethics* 10, no. 1/2 (Winter/Spring 1995): 21.

10. Michael Quint, "Health Plans Are Forcing Change in the Method for Paying Doctors," *New York Times*, 9 February 1995, A1.

11. Wendy K. Mariner, "Business vs. Medical Ethics: Conflicting Standards for Managed Care," *Journal of Law, Medicine & Ethics* 23 (1995): 246.

12. See Arthur Leibowitz et al., "Corporate Managed Care," *New England Journal of Medicine* 334, no. 16 (18 April 1996): 1060.

13. Marc A. Rodwin, *Medicine, Money, and Morals* (New York: Oxford University Press, 1993), 139–141.

14. In capitated arrangements with smaller risk pools and/or in which physician performance is tracked individually, a more direct conflict of interest occurs. In an individualized risk pool, each prescription for a test or procedure or referral to a specialist directly affects the physician's own income. Conversely, in a pool that is made up of a larger number of physicians, and in which tracking is conducted accordingly, the cost of further tests or referrals is spread throughout the group, reducing the financial importance of individual decisions. See Rodwin, *Medicine, Money, and Morals*, 139–141.

15. Ezekial J. Emanuel and Allan S. Brett, "Managed Competition and the Patient-Physician Relationship," *New England Journal of Medicine* 329, no. 12 (16 September 1993): 879–882.

16. Recently, Seagrams and other liquor manufacturers have announced that they will circumvent the industry self-imposed ban on the advertisement of liquor products on television if they can secure the air time.

17. Allan S. Brett, "The Case against Persuasive Advertising by Health Maintenance Organizations," *New England Journal of Medicine* 326, no. 20 (14 May 1992): 1353–1356.

18. William Shaw and Vincent Barry, *Moral Issues in Business*, 5th ed. (Belmont, Calif.: Wadsworth Publishing, 1992), 495–496.

19. Ronald Bayer et al., "Toward Justice in Health Care," *American Journal of Public Health* 78, no. 5 (May 1988). Reprinted in Tom L. Beauchamp

and LeRoy Walters, *Contemporary Issues in Bioethics* (Belmont, Calif.: Wadsworth Publishing, 1994), 707–715.

20. For an outstanding summary of the debate over these questions, see Beauchamp and Walters, "Justice in Access to Health Care," in *Contemporary Issues in Bioethics*, 675–682.

21. *Corcoran v United Health Care, Inc.* 965 F.2d 1321 (5th Cir. 1992).

22. Eric Larson, "The Soul of an HMO," *Time*, 26 January 1996, 48, citing Health Net medical director William Popik.

23. Marc Rodwin makes a similar argument for case managers in "Dealing with Conflicts of Interest in Managed Care," *New England Journal of Medicine* 332, no. 9 (2 March 1995): 605–607.

24. Steffie Woolhandler and David Himmelstein, Reply to Letters to the Editor, *New England Journal of Medicine* 334, no. 16 (18 April 1996): 1062.

25. Ron Winslow, "Big Buyers of Health Care Unite to Rate HMO's," *Wall Street Journal*, 3 July 1995, A3.

26. Aaron Bernstein, "Family Leave May Not Be That Big a Hardship for Business," *Business Week*, 3 June 1991, 28.

27. Michele Galen et al., "Work and Family," *Business Week*, 28 June 1993, 80–88.

28. John LaPuma et al., "Ethical Issues in Managed Care," *Trends in Health Care, Law & Ethics* 10, no. 1/2 (Winter/Spring 1995): 75.

Selected Bibliography

Abrams, Frederick R. "Caring for the Sick: An Emerging Industrial By-Product." *Journal of the American Medical Association* 255, no. 7 (21 February 1986): 937–938.

Anderson, William H. "HMO Financial Incentives and Informed Consent." *Journal of the American Medical Association* 260, no. 6 (12 August 1988): 791.

Annas, George J. "When Should Preventative Treatment Be Paid For by Health Insurance?" *New England Journal of Medicine* 331, no. 15 (13 October 1994): 1027–1030.

Archuleta, Kathleen Sutherland. "Integration of Health Care Delivery Systems: Potential Tort Liability." *Colorado Lawyer* 23, no. 8 (August 1994): 1807–1813.

Bayer, Ronald, Daniel Callahan, Arthur L. Caplan, and Bruce Jennings. "Toward Justice in Health Care." *American Journal of Public Health* 78, no. 5 (May 1988). Reprinted in Tom L. Beauchamp and LeRoy Walters, eds., *Contemporary Issues in Bioethics*, 707–715. Belmont, Calif.: Wadsworth, 1994.

Beauchamp, Tom L., and LeRoy Walters. "Justice in Access to Health Care." In *Contemporary Issues in Bioethics*, 675–682. Belmont, Calif.: Wadsworth, 1994.

Belkin, Lisa. "But What about Quality?" *New York Times Magazine*, 8 December 1996, 68–71, 101, 106.

Bernardin, Cardinal Joseph. "The Case for Not-for-Profit Health Care." Speech delivered at the Harvard Business School Club of Chicago, 12 January 1995.

Bernstein, Aaron. "Family Leave May Not Be That Big a Hardship for Business." *Business Week*, 3 June 1991, 28.

Bloom, Alan, William Ginsburg, Mark A. Kadzielski, and Kandy Waldie. "Vicarious Liability: How Vicarious and How Liable?" *Whittier Law Review* 15, no. 1 (Spring 1995): 151–176.

Bodenheimer, Thomas, and Kevin Grumbach. "The Reconfiguration of U.S. Medicine." *Journal of the American Medical Association* 274, no. 1 (5 July 1995): 85–90.

Boyle, Philip. "Business Ethics in Ethics Committees?" *Hastings Center Report* (September/October 1990): 37–38.

Brett, Allan S. "The Case against Persuasive Advertising by Health Maintenance Organizations." *New England Journal of Medicine* 326, no. 20 (14 May 1992): 1353–1356.

Brink, Susan, and Rita Rubin. "Managing Managed Care." *U.S. News & World Report*, 24 July 1995, 59–60.

Brock, Dan. "Medicine and Business: An Unhealthy Mix?" *Business and Professional Ethics Journal* 9, nos. 3&4 (1990): 21–37.

Brock, Dan W., and Allen E. Buchanan. "The Profit Motive in Medicine." *Journal of Medicine and Philosophy* 12 (1987): 1–35.

Brody, Baruch A. "Justice and Competitive Markets." *Journal of Medicine and Philosophy* 12 (1987): 37–49.

Buchanan, Allen. "Toward a Theory of the Ethics of Bureaucratic Organizations. *Business Ethics Quarterly* 6, no. 4 (October 1996): 419–440.

Burton, Brian K., and Craig P. Dunn. "Feminist Ethics As Moral Grounding for Stakeholder Theory." *Business Ethics Quarterly* 6, no. 2 (April 1996): 133–147.

California Medical Association. *Knox-Keene Health Plan Expenditures Summary: FY 1994–1995.* Sacramento: California Medical Association, February 1996.

California Medical Association. *Knox-Keene Health Plan Expenditures Summary: FY 1995–96.* Sacramento: California Medical Association, February 1997.

Callahan, Daniel. "Ethics and Priority Setting in Oregon." *Health Affairs* 10, no. 2 (Summer 1991). Reprinted in Tom L. Beauchamp and LeRoy Walters, eds., *Contemporary Issues in Bioethics,* 745–752. Belmont, Calif.: Wadsworth, 1994.

———. *Setting Limits: Medical Goals in an Aging Society.* New York: Simon & Schuster, 1987.

Cann, Ronald E. "Managed Care, Mental Health, and the Marketplace." Letter to the Editor. *Journal of the American Medical Association* 271, no. 8 (24 February 1994): 587.

Caplan, Arthur L. "Can Money and Morality Mix in Medicine?" *Academic Emergency Medicine* 1, no. 1 (1994): 73–81.

Castro, Janice. "Who Owns the Patient Anyway?" *Time,* 18 July 1994, 38–40.

The Catholic Health Association. *Setting Relationships Right: A Working Proposal for Systemic Healthcare Reform.* Washington, D.C.: The Catholic Health Association, 1992.

Chappell, Tom. *The Soul of a Business: Managing for Profit and the Common Good.* New York: Bantam, 1993.

Chassin, Mark R. "The Missing Ingredient in Health Reform: Quality of Care." *Journal of the American Medical Association* 270, no. 3 (21 July 1993): 377–378.

Child, Sherman B. "Managed Care." Letter to the Editor. *New England Journal of Medicine* 333, no. 18 (2 November 1995): 1219.

Christensen, Kate T. "Ethically Important Distinctions among Managed Care Organizations." *Journal of Law, Medicine & Ethics* 23 (1995): 223–229.

Clancy, Carolyn M., and Howard Brody. "Managed Care: Jekyll or Hyde?" *Journal of the American Medical Association* 273, no. 4 (25 January 1995): 338–339.

———. Reply to Letters to the Editor. *Journal of the American Medical Association* 274, no. 8 (23/30 August 1995): 611.

Clement, Dolores G., Sheldon M. Retchin, Randall S. Brown, and MeriBeth H. Stegall. "Access and Outcomes of Elderly Patients Enrolled in Managed Care." *Journal of the American Medical Association* 271, no. 19 (18 May 1994): 1487–1492.

Cloutier, Marc. "The Evolution of Managed Care." *Trends in Health Care, Law & Ethics* 10, no. 1/2 (Winter/Spring 1995): 67–71.

Council on Ethical and Judicial Affairs, American Medical Association. "Ethical Issues in Managed Care." *Journal of the American Medical Association* 273, no. 4 (25 January 1995): 330–335.

Cummings, Patricia J. "Third-Party Payer Tort Liability for Utilization Review Decisions." *Medical Trial Technique Quarterly* 41, no. 3 (Spring 1995): 432–453.

Daniels, Norman. "The Profit Motive and the Moral Assessment of Health Care Institutions." *Business and Professional Ethics Journal* 10, no. 2 (Summer 1991): 3–30.

Dickerson, John F. "Dr. Clinton Scrubs Up." *Time*, 8 December 1997, 48.

Donaldson, Thomas. "Constructing a Social Contract for Business." In Thomas Donaldson and Patricia A. Werhane, eds., *Ethical Issues in Business: A Philosophical Approach*, 2nd ed., 153–166. Englewood Cliffs, N.J.: Prentice-Hall, 1983.

Donaldson, Thomas, and Thomas W. Dunfee. "Toward a Unified Conception of Business Ethics: Integrative Social Contracts Theory." *Academy of Management Review* 18, no. 2 (1994): 252–284.

Donaldson, Thomas, and Lee E. Preston. "The Stakeholder Theory of the Corporation: Concepts, Evidence & Implications." *Academy of Management Review* 65 (1995): 65–91.

Dunfee, Thomas W., and Thomas Donaldson. "Contractarian Business Ethics: Current Status and Next Steps." *Business Ethics Quarterly* 5, no. 2 (April 1995): 173–186.

Eisenberg, John M. "Economics." *Journal of the American Medical Association* 273, no. 21 (7 June 1995): 1670–1671.

Ellwood, Paul M., Jr., and George D. Lundberg. "Managed Care: A Work in Progress." *Journal of the American Medical Association* 276, no. 13 (2 October 1996): 1083–1086.

Emanuel, Ezekial J. "Medical Ethics in the Era of Managed Care: The Need for Institutional Structures instead of Principles for Individual Cases." *The Journal of Clinical Ethics* 6, no. 4 (Winter 1995): 335–338.

Emanuel, Ezekial J., and Allan S. Brett. "Managed Competition and the Patient-Physician Relationship." *New England Journal of Medicine* 329, no. 12 (16 September 1993): 879–882.

Emanuel, Ezekial J., and Nancy Neveloff Dubler. "Preserving the Physician-Patient Relationship in an Era of Managed Care." *Journal of the American Medical Association* 273, no. 4 (25 January 1995): 323–329.

———. Reply to Letters to the Editor. *Journal of the American Medical Association* 274, no. 8 (23/30 August 1995): 610.

Engelhard, Carolyn Long, and James F. Childress. "Caveat Emptor: The Cost of Managed Care." *Trends in Health Care, Law & Ethics* 10, no. 1/2 (Winter/Spring 1995): 11–14, 71.

Engelhardt, H. Tristam Jr., and Michael A. Rie. "Morality for the Emerging Medical Industrial Complex." *New England Journal of Medicine* 319, no. 16 (20 October 1988): 1086–1089.

Enthoven, Alain C., and Richard Kronick. "A Consumer Choice Plan for the 1990's: Universal Health Insurance in a System Designed to Promote Quality and Economy." *New England Journal of Medicine* 320 (1988): 29–37.

———. "Universal Health Insurance through Incentives Reform." *Journal of the American Medical Association* 265, no. 19 (15 May 1991): 2532–2536.

Evan, William M., and R. Edward Freeman. "A Stakeholder Theory of the Modern Corporation: Kantian Capitalism." In Tom L. Beauchamp and Norman Bowie, eds., *Ethical Theory and Business*, 3rd ed., 97–105. Engelwood Cliffs, N.J.: Prentice-Hall, 1988.

Evans, M. Stanton, Peter L. Spencer, and Malcolm A. Kline. "The Trouble with HMO's." *Consumers' Research*, July 1995, 10–14, 34.

"Evolving Health Care System Brings New Issues." *Issues* 9, no. 5 (September/October 1994): 1–8.

Fins, Joseph. "The Hidden Costs of Market-Based Health Care Reform." *Hastings Center Report* (May–June 1992): 6.

Freeman, R. Edward. "The Business Sucks Story." Presidential address delivered at the annual meeting of the Society for Business Ethics. Vancouver, B.C., August 1995.

———. "The Politics of Stakeholder Theory: Some Future Directions." *Business Ethics Quarterly* 4 (October 1994): 409–422.

———. "A Stakeholder Theory of the Modern Corporation." In Tom L. Beauchamp and Norman E. Bowie, eds., *Ethical Theory and Business*, 5th ed., 66–76. Englewood Cliffs, N.J.: Prentice-Hall, 1997.

———. *Strategic Management: A Stakeholder Approach.* Boston: Pittman Publishing, 1984.

French, Peter. "The Corporation As a Moral Person." *American Philosophical Quarterly* 3 (1979): 207–215.

Friedman, Milton. "The Social Responsibility of Business Is to Increase Its Profits." *New York Times Magazine*, 13 September 1970, 32–33, 122–126.

Fukuyama, Francis. *Trust: The Social Virtues and the Creation of Prosperity.* New York: Free Press, 1995.

Furrow, Barry J. "Managed Care and the Evolution of Quality." *Trends in Health Care, Law & Ethics* 10, no. 1/2 (Winter/Spring 1995): 37–44.

Galen, Michele, et al. "Work and Family." *Business Week*, 28 June 1993, 80–88.

Glasson, John, and David Orentlicher. Reply to Letters to the Editor. *Journal of the American Medical Association* 274, no. 8 (23/30 August 1995): 611.

Gold, Marsha, Lyle Nelson, Timothy Lake, Robert Hurley, and Robert Berenson. "Behind the Curve: A Critical Assessment of How Little Is Known about Managed Care Plans and Physicians." *Medical Care Research & Review* 52, no. 3 (September 1995): 307–401.

Goldsmith, Jeff C., Michael Goran, and John G. Nackel. "Managed Care Comes of Age." *Healthcare Forum Journal* (September/October 1995): 14–24.

Goodman, John C., and Gerald L. Musgrave. "How to Solve the Health Care Crisis." *Consumers' Research*, March 1992, 10–14, 25.

Goodpaster, Kenneth. "Business Ethics and Stakeholder Analysis." *Business Ethics Quarterly* 1 (January 1991): 53–73.

Gosfield, Alice. "The Legal Subtext of the Managed Care Environment: A Practitioner's Perspective." *Journal of Law, Medicine & Ethics* 23 (1995): 230–235.

Gould, Brian, and Eugene D. Hill. Letter to the Editor. *Journal of the American Medical Association* 271, no. 8 (23 February 1994): 588.

Gray, Bradford H. *The Profit Motive and Patient Care: The Changing Accountability of Doctors and Hospitals*. Cambridge, Mass.: Harvard University Press, 1991.

Hadorn, David C. "The Oregon Priority-Setting Exercise: Quality of Life and Public Policy." *Hastings Center Report* 21, no. 3 (May–June 1991): 11–16.

Hasan, Malik M. "Let's End the Non-Profit Charade." *New England Journal of Medicine* 334, no. 16 (18 April 1996): 1055–1057.

Healey, William V. "The Ethics of Managed Care." *Business Ethics* (November/December 1994): 8–9.

Hiller, Marc D., and James B. Lewis. "Managed Health Care Benefit Plans: What Are the Ethical Issues?" *Trends in Health Care, Law & Ethics* 10, no. 1/2 (Winter/Spring 1995): 109–112, 118.

Hillman, Alan. "Financial Incentives for Physicians in HMO's." *New England Journal of Medicine* 317, no. 27 (1987): 1743–1749.

Hillman, Alan L., and Neil Goldfarb. "Exemplary Quality Improvement Programs in HMO's." *Journal of Quality Improvement* 21, no. 9 (September 1995): 457–464.

Hillman, Alan L., Mark V. Pauly, Keith Kerman, and Caroline Rohr Martinek. "HMO Managers' Views On Financial Incentives and Quality." *Health Affairs* (Winter 1991): 207–219.

Hillman, Alan L., Mark V. Pauly, and Joseph Kerstein. "How Do Financial Incentives Affect Physicians' Clinical Decisions and the Financial Performance of Health Maintenance Organizations?" *New England Journal of Medicine* 321, no. 2 (13 July 1989): 86–92.

Hillman, Alan L., Pete Welch, and Mark V. Pauly. "Contractual Arrangements between HMO's and Primary Care Physicians: Three Tiered HMO's and Risk Pools." *Medical Care* 30, no. 2 (February 1992): 136–148.

Hirshfield, Edward B. "Should Ethical and Legal Standards for Physicians Be Changed to Accommodate New Models for Rationing Health Care?" *University of Pennsylvania Law Review* 140 (1992): 1809–1846.

Inglehart, John K. "The American Health Care System: Managed Care." *New England Journal of Medicine* 327, no. 10 (3 September 1992): 742–747.

———. "The Struggle between Managed Care and Fee-for-Service Practice." *New England Journal of Medicine* 331, no. 1 (7 July 1994): 63–67.

Institute of Medicine. *For-Profit Enterprise in Health Care*. Edited by Bradford H. Gray. Washington, D.C.: National Academy Press, 1986.

Jackson, George S. "Adam Smith on Health Care." *Tax Notes*, 13 March 1995, 1719–1720.

Jecker, Nancy S. "Business Ethics and the Ethics of Managed Care." *Trends in Health Care, Law & Ethics* 10, no. 1/2 (Winter/Spring 1995): 53–55, 66.

———. "Managed Competition and Managed Care: What Are the Ethical Issues?" *Clinics in Geriatric Medicine* 10, no. 3 (August 1994): 527–540.

Johnson, Sandra H. "Managed Care as Regulation: Functional Ethics for a Regulated Environment." *Journal of Law, Medicine & Ethics* 23 (1995): 266–272.

Kassirer, Jerome P. "Managed Care and the Morality of the Marketplace." *New England Journal of Medicine* 333, no. 1 (6 July 1995): 50–52.

———. "The Quality of Care and the Quality of Measuring It." *New England Journal of Medicine* 329, no. 17 (21 October 1993): 1263–1265.

Kelly, Kevin, and Eric Schine. "How Did Sears Blow This Gasket?" *Business Week*, 29 June 1992, 38.

Kerr, Eve A., Brian S. Mittman, Ron D. Hays, Albert L. Siu, Barbara Leake, and Robert H. Brook. "Managed Care and Capitation in California: How Do Physicians at Financial Risk Control Their Own Utilization?" *Annals of Internal Medicine* 123 (1995): 500–504.

Kim, David E. Letter to the Editor. *New England Journal of Medicine* 333, no. 18 (2 November 1995): 1220.

Kleinke, J. D. "Triumph of the Market." *Barron's*, 24 October 1994, 59.

Kosterlitz, Julie. "Unmanaged Care?" *National Journal* (10 December 1994): 2903–2907.

Kreiger, Lloyd M. "Price and Service: A Doctor's Prescription for Managed Care." *Barron's*, 14 August 1995, 47.

Kuttner, Robert. "The Lethal Effects of Managed Care." *Business Week*, 7 August 1995, 16.

Lamm, Richard D. "Managed Care Heresies." *Trends in Health Care, Law & Ethics* 10, no. 1/2 (Winter/Spring 1995): 15–18, 72.

LaPuma, John. Letter to the Editor. *Journal of the American Medical Association* 274, no. 8 (23/30 August 1995): 610.

LaPuma, John, David Schiedermayer, and Mark Seigler. "Ethical Issues in Managed Care." *Trends in Health Care, Law & Ethics* 10, no. 1/2 (Winter/Spring 1995): 73–77, 96.

Larson, David. "Business and Medicine: Are They Ethically Compatible?" *Update* 7, no. 3 (September 1991). In Lisa Newton and Maureen Ford, eds., *Taking Sides: Business and Society*, 3rd ed., 49–54. Guilford, Conn.: Dushkin Publishing Group, 1994.

Larson, Erik. "The Soul of an HMO." *Time*, 22 January 1996, 45–52.

Leibowitz, Arthur, Nicholas A. Hanchak, and Neil Schlackman. "Corporate Managed Care." Letter to the Editor. *New England Journal of Medicine* 334, no. 16 (18 April 1996): 1060.

Lewis, Randall J. Letter to the Editor. *New England Journal of Medicine* 333, no. 18 (2 November 1995): 1220.

Macklin, Ruth. *Enemies of Patients*. New York: Oxford University Press, 1993.

———. "The Ethics of Managed Care." *Trends in Health Care, Law & Ethics* 10, no. 1/2 (Winter/Spring 1995): 63–66.

"Managed Care Brings a Demand for Institutional Ethics Policies." *Medical Ethics Advisor* 10, no. 10 (October 1994): 127–128.

Margolis, Joshua D. "Casting Business As a Profession." Paper presented at the 1996 annual meeting of the Society for Business Ethics. Quebec City, August 1996.

Mariner, Wendy K. "Business vs. Medical Ethics: Conflicting Standards for Managed Care." *Journal of Law, Medicine & Ethics* 23 (1995): 236–246.

Maxwell, Thomas J. "Health Reform/Managed Care: A View from a Doctor's Office." *Delaware Lawyer* (Spring 1995): 34–40.

May, William W. "Managed Care: Insurers, Values, and the Bottom Line on Care." Paper presented at the American Academy of Religion, New Orleans, 25 November 1996.

McCormick, Brian. "Law Thwarts Physician Networks." *American Medical News* 38, no. 33 (4 September 1995): 1.

———. "Managed Care Posing New Liability Risks, Insurers Warn." *American Medical News* 37, no. 22 (13 June 1994): 3–7.

McGarvey, Michael. "The Case for Managed Care." *Trends in Health Care, Law & Ethics* 10, no. 1/2 (Winter/Spring 1995): 45–46, 52.

Mechanic, David. "Professional Judgment and the Rationing of Medical Care." *University of Pennsylvania Law Review* 140 (1992): 1713–1754.

Mehlman, Maxwell J., and Susan R. Massey. "The Patient-Physician Relationship and the Allocation of Scarce Resources: A Law and Economics Approach." *Kennedy Institute of Ethics Journal* 4, no. 4 (1994): 291–308.

Menzel, Paul T. "Economic Competition in Health Care: A Moral Assessment." *Journal of Medicine and Philosophy* 12 (1987): 63–84.

Merline, John W. "Making Money by Denying Care." *Consumers' Research*, September 1994, 10–15.

Miller, Robert H., and Harold S. Luft. "Managed Care Plan Performance since 1980: A Literature Analysis." *Journal of the American Medical Association* 271, no. 19 (18 May 1994): 1512–1519.

"Mismanaged Care." *American Medical News* 38, no. 118 (8 May 1995): 27.

Moffit, Robert Emmet. "Personal Freedom and Responsibility: The Ethical Foundations of a Market-Based Health Care Reform System." *Journal of Medicine and Philosophy* 19, no. 5 (October 1995): 471–481.

Morreim, E. Haavi. *Balancing Act: The New Medical Ethics of Medicine's New Economics.* Dordrecht, The Netherlands: Kluwer Academic Publishers, 1991.

———. "Cost Containment: Challenging Fidelity and Justice." *Hastings Center Report* (December 1988): 20–25.

———. "Moral Justice and Legal Justice in Managed Care: The Ascent of Contributive Justice." *Journal of Law, Medicine & Ethics* 23 (1995): 247–265.

Munn, Randall. "Managed Care/Utilization Review Liability." *Nevada Lawyer* 17, no. 1 (August 1993): 23–27.

Newton, Lisa, and Maureen Ford. "Postscript: Are Business and Medicine Ethically Compatible?" In Newton and Ford, eds., *Taking Sides: Business and Society*, 3rd ed., 55. Guilford, Conn.: Dushkin Publishing Group, 1994.

Novak, Michael. *Business as a Calling.* New York: Free Press, 1996.

———. *The Spirit of Democratic Capitalism.* Lantham, Md.: Madison Books/University Press of America, 1991.

———. *This Hemisphere of Liberty.* Washington, D.C.: AEI Press, 1992.

Nudelman, Phillip M., and Linda M. Andrews. "The 'Value-Added' of Not-for-Profit Health Plans." *New England Journal of Medicine* 334, no. 16 (18 April 1996): 1057–1059.

Orentlicher, David. "Managed Care and the Threat to the Patient-Physician Relationship." *Trends in Health Care, Law & Ethics* 10, no. 1/2 (Winter/Spring 1995): 19–24.

———. "Physician Advocacy for Patients under Managed Care." *The Journal of Clinical Ethics* 6, no. 4 (Winter 1995): 333–334.

Page, Leigh. "Market Spawns Doctor-Patient Alliances." *American Medical News* 38, no. 42 (13 November 1995): 3.

Paine, Lynne Sharp. "Managing for Organizational Integrity." *Harvard Business Review* (March–April 1994): 106–117.

Parmet, Wendy E. "The Impact of Health Insurance Reform on the Law Governing the Physician-Patient Relationship." *Journal of the American Medical Association* 268, no. 24 (23/30 December 1992): 3468–3472.

Pellegrino, Edmund D. "Allocation of Resources at the Bedside: The Intersections of Economics, Law, and Ethics." *Kennedy Institute of Ethics Journal* 4, no. 4 (1994): 309–317.

———. "Ethics." *Journal of the American Medical Association* 271, no. 21 (1 June 1994): 1668–1670.

———. "Interests, Obligations, and Justice: Some Notes toward an Ethic of Managed Care." *Journal of Clinical Ethics* 6, no. 4 (Winter 1995): 312–317.

———. "Toward a Virtue-Based Normative Ethics for the Health Care Professions." *Kennedy Institute of Ethics Journal* 5, no. 3 (1995): 253–277.

———. "Words Can Hurt You: Some Reflections on the Metaphors of Managed Care." First Annual Nicholas J. Pisano Lecture. *Journal of the American Board of Family Practice* 7, no. 6 (November–December 1994): 505–510.

Phillips, Robert A. "Stakeholder Theory and A Principle of Fairness." *Business Ethics Quarterly* 7, no. 1 (January 1997): 51–66.

Praeger, Linda O. "State Licensing Boards Consider Curbing Financial Incentives." *American Medical News* 38, no. 39 (16 October 1995): 1.

Rabkin, Mitchell T. "Control of Healthcare Costs: Targeting and Coordinating the Incentives." *New England Journal of Medicine* 309, no. 16 (20 October 1993): 982–984.

Rainbolt, George W. "Competition and the Patient-Centered Ethic." *Journal of Medicine and Philosophy* 12 (1987): 85–99.

Rawls, John. *Political Liberalism.* New York: Columbia University Press, 1993.

———. *A Theory of Justice.* Cambridge, Mass.: Harvard University Press, 1971.

Reinhardt, Uwe E. "Breaking American Health Policy Gridlock." *Health Affairs* (Summer 1991): 96–103.

———. "Health Reform is Dead! Long Live Health Reform!" *Trends in Health Care, Law & Ethics* 10, no. 1/2 (Winter/Spring 1995): 7–10, 32.

———. "Managed Competition in Health Care Reform: Just Another American Dream, or the Perfect Solution?" *Journal of Law, Medicine & Ethics* 22, no. 2 (Summer 1994): 106–120.

Relman, Arnold S. "Medical Practice under the Clinton Reforms: Avoiding Domination by Big Business." *New England Journal of Medicine* 329, no. 21 (18 November 1993): 1574–1576.

———. "What About Managed Care?" *New England Journal of Medicine* 331, no. 7 (18 August 1994): 471–472.

———. "What Market Values Are Doing to Medicine." *Atlantic Monthly*, March 1992, 98–106.

Relman, Arnold and Uwe Reinhardt. "An Exchange on For-Profit Health Care." Institute of Medicine, *For-Profit Enterprise in Health Care*, ed. Bradford H. Gray, 209–223. Washington, D.C.: National Academy Press, 1986.

Rilmer, George W., and Richard D. Morrison. "The Ethical Impacts of Managed Care." *Journal of Business Ethics* 12, no. 6 (June 1993): 493–501.

Rivoli, Pietra. "Ethical Aspects of Investor Behavior." *Journal of Business Ethics* 14, no. 4 (April 1995): 265–277.

Rodwin, Marc A. "Dealing with Conflicts of Interest in Managed Care." *New England Journal of Medicine* 332, no. 9 (2 March 1995): 605–607.

———. *Medicine, Money, and Morals.* New York: Oxford University Press, 1993.

Rooney, J. Patrick. "Medisave in Practice: An Insurer's Example." *Consumers' Research*, March 1992, 12–13.

Rubin, Rita. "Rating the HMO's." *U.S. News & World Report*, 2 September 1996, 52–55.

Safran, Dana Gelb, Alvin R. Tarlov, and William H. Rogers. "Primary Care Performance in Fee-for-Service and Prepaid Health Care Systems." *Journal of the American Medical Association* 271, no. 20 (25 May 1994): 1579–1586.

Salmon, John G. "Litigating Claims against Managed Health Care Organizations." *Trial* (February 1995): 80–85.

Schindler, Thomas. "Considerations in Managed Care." *Health Progress* (December 1994): 52–55.

Schmidt, Charles E., Jr. "Managed Care Faces Stinging Backlash." *Best's Review* (November 1995): 21–23, 84–86.

Scofield, Giles R. "Mangled Care." *Trends in Health Care, Law & Ethics* 10, no. 1/2 (Winter/Spring 1995): 47–51.

Shaw, William, and Vincent Barry. *Moral Issues in Business*, 5th ed. Belmont, Calif.: Wadsworth Publishing, 1992, 202–209.

Shepard, Jon M., James C. Wimbush, and Carroll U. Stephens. "The Place of Ethics in Business: Shifting Paradigms." *Business Ethics Quarterly* 5, no. 3 (July 1995): 577–601.

Shore, Miles F., and Harry Levinson. "On Business and Medicine." *New England Journal of Medicine* 313, no. 5 (1 August 1985): 319–321.

Smith, H. R., and Archie B. Carroll. "Organizational Ethics: A Stacked Deck." *Journal of Business Ethics* 3 (1984): 95–100.

Solomon, Gil L. "Length of the Hospital Stay for Newborn Mothers." Letter to the Editor. *New England Journal of Medicine* 334, no. 17 (25 April 1996): 1134.

Solomon, Robert. *Ethics and Excellence: Cooperation and Integrity in Business.* New York: Oxford University Press, 1992.

Starfield, Barbara, Neil R. Rowe, Jonathan Weiner, Mary Stuart, Donald Steinwachs, Sarah Hudson Scholle, and Andrea Gertensberger. "Cost vs. Quality in Different Types of Primary Care Settings." *Journal of the American Medical Association* 272, no. 24 (28 December 1994): 1903–1908.

Stock, Howard. Letter to the Editor. *Journal of the American Medical Association* 271, no. 8 (23 February 1994): 588.

Stodghill, Ron, II, Eric Schine, and Joseph Weber. "Sudden Illness: Managed Care Faces a Harsh New Reality." *Business Week*, 8 May 1995, 32–33.

Stone, Alan A. "Law's Influence on Medicine and Medical Ethics." *New England Journal of Medicine* 312, no. 5 (31 January 1985): 309–312.

Sugar, Sam J. Letter to the Editor. *New England Journal of Medicine* 333, no. 18 (2 November 1995): 1220.

Tanner, Michael. "Returning Medicine to the Marketplace." In David Boaz and Edward Crane, eds., *Market Liberalism: A Paradigm for the 21st Century*. Washington, D.C.: Cato Institute, 1993.

Taylor, Amy K., Karen M. Beauregard, and Jessica P. Vistnes. "Who Belongs to HMO's: A Comparison of Fee-for-Service versus HMO Enrollees." *Medical Care Research and Review* 52, no. 3 (September 1995): 389–408.

Tenery, Robert M., Jr. "Competition May Ensure Quality in Managed Care." *American Medical News* 38, no. 17 (1 May 1995): 25–26.

Thomasma, David C. "The Ethics of Managed Care and Cost Control." *Trends in Health Care, Law & Ethics* 10, no. 1/2 (Winter/Spring 1995): 33–36, 41.

Thompson, Dennis J. "Understanding Financial Conflicts of Interest." *Journal of the American Medical Association* 329, no. 8 (19 August 1993): 573–576.

Thorpe, Kenneth E. "Medical Savings Accounts: Design and Policy Issues." *Health Affairs* 14, no. 3 (1995): 254–259.

Velasquez, Manuel. "Why Corporations Are Not Morally Responsible for Anything They Do." *Business & Professional Ethics Journal* 2 (Spring 1983): 8.

Vladeck, Bruce C. "Managed Care and Quality." *Journal of the American Medical Association* 273, no. 19 (17 May 1995): 1483.

Wagner, Edward. "The Cost-Quality Relationship: Do We Always Get What We Pay For?" *Journal of the American Medical Association* 272, no. 24 (28 December 1994): 1951–1952.

Ware, John E., Martha Bayliss, William H. Rogers, Mark Kosinski, and Alvin R. Tarlov. "Differences in 4-Year Health Outcomes for Elderly and Poor, Chronically Ill Patients Treated in HMO and Fee-for-

Service Systems: Results from the Medical Outcomes Study." *Journal of the American Medical Association* 276, no. 13 (2 October 1996): 1039–1047.

Waymack, Mark H. "Health Care as a Business: The Ethic of Hippocrates versus the Ethic of Managed Care." *Business and Professional Ethics Journal* 9, nos. 3&4 (1990): 69–78.

Weidenbaum, Murray. "Can the Free Market Cure America's Health Care Disease?" *Business and Society Review* 93 (Spring 1995): 26–32.

Weil, Thomas P. "Managed Health Care: A Utility Style Monopoly?" *Public Utilities Fortnightly*, 1 February 1995, 14–15.

Werhane, Patricia H. *Adam Smith and His Legacy for Modern Capitalism*. New York: Oxford University Press, 1991.

———. "The Ethics of Health Care As a Business." *Business and Professional Ethics Journal* 9, nos. 3&4 (1990): 7–20.

———. "The Ethics of Insider Trading." *Journal of Business Ethics* 8 (1989): 841–845.

White, Jane. "Health System Changes in the Absence of National Reform." *Health Progress*, December 1994, 10–16.

Wicks, Andrew C. "Albert Schweitzer or Ivan Boesky? Why We Should Reject the Dichotomy between Medicine and Business." *Journal of Business Ethics* 14, no. 5 (May 1995): 339–351.

———. "The Business Ethics Movement: Where Are We Headed and What Can We Learn from Our Colleagues in Bioethics?" *Business Ethics Quarterly* 5, no. 3 (1995): 603–620.

———. "Overcoming the Separation Thesis: The Need for Reconsideration of Business and Society Research." *Business and Society* 35, no. 1 (March 1996): 89–118.

Wolf, Susan M. "Health Care Reform and the Future of Physician Ethics." *Hastings Center Report* 24, no. 2 (1994): 28–41.

———. "Quality Assessment of Ethics in Health Care: The Accountability Revolution." *American Journal of Law & Medicine* 20, no. 1/2 (1994): 105–128.

———. "Toward a Theory of Process." *Law, Medicine & Health Care* 20, no. 4 (Winter 1992): 278–290.

Wolinsky, Howard. "Ethics in Managed Care." *The Lancet* 345 (10 June 1995): 1499.

Woodstock Theological Center, Seminar in Business Ethics. *Ethical Considerations in the Business Aspects of Health Care*. Washington, D.C.: Georgetown University Press, 1995.

Wooley, Susan, Michele Galen, Ann Therese Palmer, Joan O. C. Hamilton, and Chris Rousch. "Physician, Restrain Thyself." *Business Week*, 13 September 1993, 32–33.

Woolhandler, Steffie, and David Himmelstein. Reply to Letters to the Editor. *New England Journal of Medicine* 334, no. 16 (18 April 1996): 1062.

Zwerner, Alan. Letter to the Editor. *New England Journal of Medicine* 334, no. 16 (18 April 1996): 1061–1062.

NEWSPAPER ARTICLES

Anders, George, and Laura Johannes. "Doctors Are Losing a Lobbying Battle to HMO's." *Wall Street Journal*, 15 May 1995, B1.

"An Anti-Patient Act." *New York Times*, 31 May 1995, A20 (L).

Bristow, Lonnie R. "Let's Not Rule Out Managed Care Accounts." Letter to the Editor. *New York Times*, 9 October 1995, A10(N).

Broder, David S. "Managed Care Savings Seen." *Washington Post*, 12 May 1994, A9.

Broder, Michael S. "In Health Care, We Cannot Have It All." *Los Angeles Times*, 27 December 1995, B9.

"Doctors Sue Aetna over HMO Treatment Policy." *Los Angeles Times*, 23 August 1995, D3.

Dowling, Katherine. "Medicine from the Factory Line." *Los Angeles Times*, 2 August 1995, B9.

Elias, Paul. "Trial No Longer a Managed Care Test." *Los Angeles Times*, 10 November 1995, A3.

Enthoven, Alain C. "In Defense of Managed Care." Letter to the Editor. *Wall Street Journal*, 17 February 1994, A17(E).

Enthoven, Alain C., and Richard Kronick. "Better Medicine at Lower Cost." *New York Times*, 12 June 1994, HR 6 (L).

Enthoven, Alain C., and Sara J. Singer. "2010 Will Be Too Late to Reform." *Los Angeles Times*, 12 March 1997, B3.

Flannigan, James. "The Changing State of Managed Care." *Los Angeles Times*, 23 June 1996, D1.

Freudenheim, Milton. "To Economists, Managed Care Is No Cure-All." *New York Times*, 6 September 1994, A1.

Goldsmith, Oliver. "HMO Revolution in California." Letter to the Editor. *Los Angeles Times*, 6 September 1995, B8.

Goodman, John C. "A Plan to Empower Patients." *Wall Street Journal*, 2 May 1995, A24.

Goodman, Walter. "The Complexities of Managed Care." *New York Times*, 6 September 1995, C16.

Gordon, Suzanne. "Hippocratic or Hypocratic Oath?" *Los Angeles Times*, 21 January 1996, M5.

———. "A 'Quicker and Sicker' Rebellion." *Los Angeles Times*, 23 July 1995, M5.

Gordon, Suzanne, and Ellen D. Baer. "Keeping Quiet on the Tough Choices." *Los Angeles Times*, 24 January 1995, B7.

Hiltzik, Michael A. "Drawing the Line: An HMO Dilemma." *Los Angeles Times*, 17 January 1996, A1.

———. "Health Insurers' Growing Clout Stirs Concerns." *Los Angeles Times*, 3 July 1995, A1.

———. "HMO Slapped with $1-Million Judgment in Cancer Case." *Los Angeles Times*, 18 October 1996, D1.

———. "Supreme Court Won't Allow Suit in Death Case." *Los Angeles Times*, 16 May 1995, D1.

Hiltzik, Michael A., and David Olmos. "A Mixed Diagnosis for HMO's." *Los Angeles Times*, 7 August 1995, A1.

"HMO Mergers Threaten to Bleed Competition." *Los Angeles Times*, 23 January 1997, B8.

"How HMO Expenses Break Down." *Los Angeles Times*, 15 February 1996, D2.

Krieger, Lloyd M. "How Managed Care Will Allow Market Forces to Solve the Problems." *New York Times*, 13 August 1995, F12(L).

Lamb, David. "Massachusetts Mill Town Gets Angel for Christmas." *Los Angeles Times*, 19 December 1995, A24.

Lawrence, David. "The Market Is Already Doing It." *Wall Street Journal*, 16 March 1994, A18.

Levine, Bettijane. "He Might Have the Cure for Medicine's Ills." *Los Angeles Times*, 18 July 1995, E1.

"Lost in the HMO Maze." *Los Angeles Times*, 3 October 1996, B8.

"Managed Care Providers Where Doctors Used to Be." *Washington Post*, 27 June 1995, WH6.

Marmor, Theodore R., and Jerry L. Mashaw. "Madison Ave. Meets Marcus Welby." *Los Angeles Times*, 19 February 1995, M5.

McCombs, Jeff. "Health Care." Letter to the Editor. *Los Angeles Times*, 8 January 1996, B4.

Mittermaier, Alan. "Give Your HMO a Thorough Annual Checkup." *Wall Street Journal*, October 1995, A12(E).

Mittler, Brant S. "The Myth of Unnecessary Care." *Wall Street Journal*, 1 March 1993, A14.

Morain, Claudia. "Looking for More Controls in Managed Care in California." *American Medical News* 38, no. 18 (8 May 1995): 5–6.

"New Hope for HMO Patients Who Have Precious Little." *Los Angeles Times*, 29 August 1996, B8.

"Nonprofit Accrediting Group Releases HMO Performance Data." *Los Angeles Times*, 22 August 1996, D2.

Olmos, David R. "As Cutbacks Hit Limit, Health Costs Rise Anew." *Los Angeles Times*, 16 April 1997, A1.

———. "Blue Shield, in Bold Move, Will Waive Specialist Referrals." *Los Angeles Times*, 18 June 1996, D1.

———. "California Care Scores Poorly in Quality Review." *Los Angeles Times*, 5 October 1995, D6.

———. "Cutting Health Costs or Corners?" *Los Angeles Times*, 5 May 1995, A1.

———. "Dueling HMO Reform Plans Vie for Votes." *Los Angeles Times*, 7 October 1996, A1.

———. "Elderly and Poor Fare Worse in HMO's, Study Says." *Los Angeles Times*, 2 October 1996, A1.

———. "HMO Cites $20 Million in Failed-Merger Costs." *Los Angeles Times*, 13 February 1996, D3.

———. "HMO's Shut Out of Latest Health Care Trend." *Los Angeles Times*, 27 October 1996, A1.

———. "HMO's Vary in Preventive Care, Study Says." *Los Angeles Times*, 26 June 1996, D2.

———. "Kaiser Seeking to Pay Bonuses to Nurses Who Help Cut Costs." *Los Angeles Times*, 22 December 1995, D1.

———. "Law Will Boost Terminal Patient's Rights." *Los Angeles Times*, 28 September 1996, A22.

———. "Members Like Small HMO's Best, Poll Says." *Los Angeles Times*, 12 September 1996, D2.

———. "Search for a Fraud Cure: Federal Task Force Is Looking into Abuse in Managed Care Field." *Los Angeles Times*, 18 March 1995, D1+.

———. "2 Plans to Regulate HMO's Move toward Ballot." *Los Angeles Times*, 23 April 1996, A21.

Olmos, David R., and Michael Hiltzik. "Doctors Authority, Pay Dwindle under HMO's." *Los Angeles Times*, 29 August 1995, A1.

Olmos, David R., and Shari Roan. "HMO Gag Clauses on Doctors Spur Protest." *Los Angeles Times*, 14 April 1996, A1.

Pear, Robert. "H.M.O's Refusing Emergency Claims, Hospitals Assert." *New York Times*, 9 July 1995, A1.

Price, Westcott, III. "Managed Care Now; It Works." *Los Angeles Times*, 14 March 1995, B7.

Quint, Michael. "Health Plans Are Forcing Change in the Method for Paying Doctors." *New York Times*, 5 February 1995, A1.

Ramsey, Bruce. "Medical Savings Accounts Turn Out to Be Hard Sell." *Seattle Post-Intelligencer*, 24 September 1997, E1.

Rich, Spence. "Doctors Pay Drops to Average of 186,600 in 1994 Due to Managed Care." *Washington Post*, 3 September 1996, A13.

Rosenblatt, Robert A. "Doctors, HMO's Clash at Hearing 'Gag Rules'." *Los Angeles Times*, 31 May 1996, A1.

———. "Doctors Prescribe Medicare HMO's as Panacea for Ailing Bottom Lines." *Los Angeles Times*, 25 November 1995, A29.

———. "Federal Mandates in Health Insurance Alarm Providers." *Los Angeles Times*, 3 October 1996, D1.

———. "Medicare HMO's Told They Cannot Gag Physicians." *Los Angeles Times*, 7 December 1996, A1.

———. "Republicans Devise Plan to Cap Open-Ended Medicare Outlays." *Los Angeles Times*, 19 July 1995, A5.

Rosenblatt, Robert A., and Edwin Chen. "AMA Backs GOP Medicare Plan." *Los Angeles Times*, 11 October 1995, A1+.

Schachter, Jim. "Insured People Satisfied with Medical Care." *Los Angeles Times*, 28 August 1995, A1.

Segal, David. "Health Care Costs Hit Milestone." *Washington Post*, 28 September 1995, D13.

Sharpe, Anita, "How 'Medicaid Moms' Became a Hot Market for Health Industry." *Wall Street Journal*, 1 May 1997, A1.

Shuit, Douglas P. "State Medical Association to Cite High Cost of Private Health Plans." *Los Angeles Times*, 18 April 1995, A3.

Skrzycki, Cindy. "Doctors Lobby Congress in Tug of War over Patients." *Washington Post*, 6 October 1995, F1.

Smith, Lynn. "When Did They Take the 'Care' Out of 'Health Care'?" *Los Angeles Times*, 6 April 1997, E3.

Steinmetz, Greg. "Metlife Probed in Several States for Sales Tactics." *Wall Street Journal*, Eastern ed., 6 January 1994, B1.

Stoker, Michael. "The Ticket to Better Managed Care." *New York Times*, 28 October 1995, 21(L).

Stolberg, Sheryl. "Dole's Push for Health Savings Accounts Defeated." *Los Angeles Times*, 19 April 1996, A1.

Sullivan, Joseph. "Officials Scrutinizing Doctor Bonuses in Managed Care Plans." *New York Times*, 21 September 1995, B6(L).

"Unmuzzling HMO Physicians." *Los Angeles Times*, 2 July 1996, B6.

Vladeck, Bruce. "Medicare Has No Use for Managed Care." *New York Times*, 14 June 1995, A24(L).

Walters, Donna K. H. "Californians' Raises Are the Lowest in 25 Years, Survey Says." *Los Angeles Times*, 19 July 1995, D1.

Winslow, Ron. "AMA Sets Up Program to Help Doctors Fund Their Own Managed-Care Plans." *Wall Street Journal*, 15 Feburary 1995, B6.

———. "Big Buyers of Health Care Unite to Rate HMO's." *Wall Street Journal*, 3 July 1995, A3.

———. "Employer Costs Slip As Workers Shift to HMO's." *Wall Street Journal*, 14 February 1995, A3.

———. "Employer Group Rethinks Commitment to Big HMO's." *Wall Street Journal*, 21 July 1995, B1(E).

Zaremburg, Alan. "Costs, Benefits of Managed Care." Letter to the Editor. *Los Angeles Times*, 17 September 1995, M4.

Index

Health Systems International, 20, 50, 115
Hippocratic Oath, 1, 18
hiring practices, 104
HMOs. *See* health maintenance organiza-
    tions (HMOs)
hospital bed occupancy, 121

iatrogenic harm, 49–50
implicit rationing, 44–45, 88, 92, 95
incentives. *See* financial incentives
Independent Practice Associations (IPAs),
    18, 95
indigent health care, 72, 112–14, 149
infertility treatments, 75
information disclosure, 24, 135, 144–45,
    148, 149
informed consent, 36, 82–83, 144
Inglehart, John K., 69
injury, ranking for rationing, 43
Institute of Medicine study, 73
institutional culpability, 137
institutional ethics, 6
insurance plans, choices offered, 119
insurance premiums
    costs of, 12
    inflation rates compared to, 52, 64
    rate of increase, 51
    stability of, 121
investigative procedures clauses, 18, 145
IPAs. *See* Independent Practice Associations
    (IPAs)

Jecker, Nancy, 75, 142
Johnson, Sandra, 76–77
Johnson and Johnson, 132
Journal of the American Medical Association, on
    shareholder profits, 55
justice, principles of, 7–8, 84, 140–41, 155

Kaiser-Permanente
    cost-cutting practices, 107
    doctor ratio of, 49
    and drive-through deliveries, 17, 22
    medical-loss ratio of, 109
    as prepaid care precursor, 12
    in satisfaction survey, 111
    as staff model organization, 14, 56, 110
Kassirer, Jerome, 22, 35
kickbacks, from hospitals, 67
Kronick, Richard, 58

laissez-faire model, 3, 63, 130
La Puma, John, 78
large-scale organizations, 34

lawsuits, 15–16, 17–18, 26–27. *See also* mal-
    practice suits
legislation
    for anti-trust relief, 57
    cautions on restrictive, 154
    corporate constituency statutes, 132
    current environment, 23–28
    on post-birth hospital stays, 17
    reform such as Patient Protection Act,
        23–24, 54, 69
    for utilization review, 151
    any-willing-provider provisions, 37
Lewin-VHI Inc., 95
liberty-based perspectives, 52–53
Lifeguard, 111
Los Angeles Times
    on California managed care, 66
    on corporate greed, 66
    on satisfaction rates, 53

McGarvey, Michael, 50
malpractice suits. *See also* lawsuits
    avoidance of, 22
    MCO liability, 24–25
managed care
    advocacy of, 2, 3
    background, 12–14
    best features of, 47
    case for cautious support, 121–24
    case for morality of, 93–96
    cautious supporters of, 57–59
    common arguments in support, 47–50
    concept *vs.* organizational form, 55, 57
    criticism of, 32–37
    debate perspectives, 29–32
    delivery, 7
    ethical issues, 7–8, 14–18
    for-profit champions, 50–54, 115–21
    and implicit rationing, 92, 95
    market forces on, 63
    metaphors of, 35
    moral typology, 30–32
    MSAs combined with, 87
    profit motive, 31, 32
    as rationing scheme, 34
managed care organizations
    complaints against, 51
    conflict of financial goals and service
        methods, 123–24
    contributions of, 22
    cost-saving mechanisms, 35–36
    as dominant health care delivery
        model, 141–42
    ethical framework, 122–23

Oregon Medicaid plan, 3, 43, 45, 91
Orentlicher, David, 88, 92, 146
out-of-network services, 12

Pacific Business Group on Health, 111
patient bill of rights, 23
patient-centered ethic, 68–71, 94, 95
patient-centered purists
    about, 32–37
    and fee-for-service systems, 61–62, 63,
        65, 74, 78–79
patient-physician relationship. *See* physician-patient relationship
Patient Protection Act, 23–24, 54, 69
patients
    as cost-unconscious consumers, 48
    health and profit motive, 117
    market incentives for, 38–39
    medical awareness of, 82–83, 118–19,
        153–54
    as shoppers and negotiators, 83–85
    as reasonable consumers, 94
    responsibilities of, 153–54
    satisfaction rates of, 53, 111, 116–17
Pellegrino, Edmund, 19, 35, 133
performance measurement tools, 145
physician-patient relationship
    interference in, 14, 38
    and managed care, 36
    prevailing assumptions, 77–78
physicians
    and altruism, 66–68, 128
    capitation-basis remuneration, 76–77
    ethical standards, 21
    financially motivated behavior, 66–68,
        77, 128, 133–34
    gag orders on, 16–17, 18
    as gatekeepers, 15, 21
    profit motive pressures on, 55
    refusal of Medicare patients, 66–67
    remuneration of, 15, 50
    returns on investment, 102
    salary levels of, 68
Pisano, Susan, 22
plan contract term disclosure, 144–45
point-of-service options, 24
Political Liberalism (Rawls), 7–8
poor patients
    as community responsibility, 149
    in HMO settings, 72
    in non-profit settings, 112–14
portability issues, 41, 120
post-birth hospital stays, 17, 22

preexisting conditions, 75, 120
premiums. *See* insurance premiums
prepaid group practice, 12
prepaid medical care programs, history
    of, 12
preventative care
    monitoring quality of, 148
    in shareholder-owned organizations, 122
    skimping on, 108, 120, 151–52
profit motive
    advocacy of, 50–51
    and managed care, 31, 32
    and patient health, 18–20, 117
    pressures on physicians, 55
profits, as savings to consumers, 64

quality-of-life assessments, 43–44
quality standards and measurement, 51–52,
    71–74, 121–22, 145–46, 149, 153

Rand Corporation, 39, 48, 73, 101
rationing. *See also* explicit rationers
    about, 42–45
    bedside, 56, 88
    dangerous criteria of, 89, 90
    implicit, 44–45, 88, 92, 95
    models of, 3, 7, 92
    presence of, 75
    priorities, 45, 89, 90–92
    by sin exclusion, 43, 89, 90
Rawls, John
    principles of justice, 7–8, 84, 131, 140–
        41, 144, 155
    preservation of liberty, 93
referrals, financial motivation for, 67–68
Reinhardt, Uwe, 7, 52, 66, 68–69, 102, 114
Relman, Arnold, 55, 57, 74, 102, 135
remuneration
    capitation basis, 76–77
    of physicians, 15, 50
    three-tier model of, 76
respondeat superior doctrine, 25
responsibilities
    of community, 149–52
    of employers, 152–53
    governmental, 149–52
    of managed care organizations, 143–49
    moral, 6, 99–102, 137–38
    of patients, 153–54
    social, 131
restrained market approach, 57
review organizations, 151
Rie, Michael, 52–53, 54, 117

risk pools, 147–48
risk sharing, 148–49
Rivoli, Pietra, 129

Safran, Dana, 72
satisfaction rates, 53, 111, 116–17
Scofield, Giles, 69
self-interest, greed distinct from, 126–28
separation thesis, 128–29, 140
shareholder-owned organizations
  and market discipline, 116
  quality measures and monitoring systems, 121–22
shareholders
  dividends to, 109
  financial contributions of, 130
  profits of, 55–56, 57
  social concerns of, 129
  vs. stakeholders, 62
sin-exclusion rationing, 43, 89, 90
skimming economic cream, 19, 53, 66–67, 99, 112–13
Smith, Adam, 120, 125, 126–29, 132, 149
social concerns, of shareholders, 129
socialized medicine, 113, 134
social responsibilities, 131
"The Social Responsibility of Business Is to Increase Its Profits" (Friedman), 125
specialists
  copayment bypasses of, 122
  increase in numbers, 121
  use without gatekeeper approval, 65
staff model organizations, 14, 18, 56, 110
stakeholder approach, 130–33, 136–38, 141–42, 154–55
stakeholders, vs. shareholders, 62
standards
  ethical, for physicians, 21
  for expenditure reporting, 110
  minimum for health care, 150–51
  of quality, 51–52, 71–74, 121–22
Starbucks, 132
Starfield, Barbara, 73

studies
  on financial incentives, 39
  on health maintenance organizations, 63–64
  on Medicare, 73
  methodological weaknesses, 110
  on quality of care, 72–74
  on wasteful medical procedures, 48
Swedish care model, 113, 134

tax incentives, for waste reduction, 40
tax status, of organizations, 57, 103, 116
technology, legislation outpaced by, 27
Texas Business Group, 54
A Theory of Justice (Rawls), 7–8
Theory of Moral Sentiments (Smith), 126
Thomasma, David, 23, 93
Thorpe, Kenneth, 84, 86
triple-option plans, 122
turnover rates, of insureds, 151
two realms problem, 128–29, 140

uniform regulations, lack of, 119
United Healthcare, 71–72
U.S. HealthCare, 122
utilization review, 24, 25, 146, 151

Virginia Board of Health Professions, 72

Ware, John, 72
waste
  with free goods, 101
  in medical procedure, 48
  in spending, 146
  tax incentives for reduction, 40
watchdog function, 127
Waymack, Mark, 53, 117–18
Wealth of Nations (Smith), 126
WellPoint Health Network, 20
Werhane, Patricia, 126, 127, 139–40
Wicks, Andrew, 125, 127, 129, 132, 139–40
Wolf, Susan, 4–5